Professional Practice for Physician Assistants

Elyse Watkins, DHSc, PA-C, DFAAPA

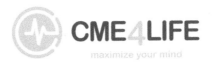

CME 4 LIFE
maximize your mind

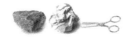

RPSS Publishing - Buffalo, New York

publisher@rockpapersafetyscissors.com

ISBN: 978-1-7326830-1-3
Printed in the United States of America

10 9 8 7 6 5 4 3 2 1

CONTENTS

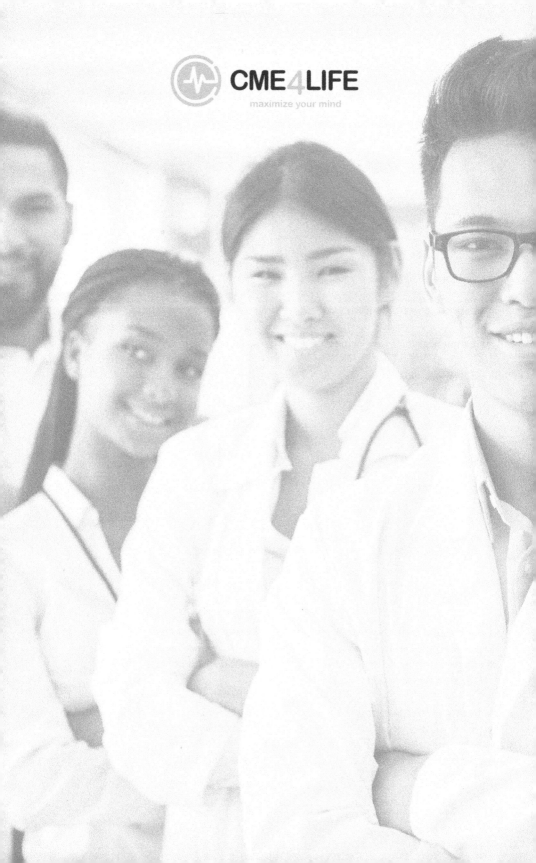

FOREWORD

The practice of medicine, as a physician assistant, is much more than antibiotics, pathophysiology of disease and physical exams. Sure, we need foundations; we need building blocks, yet to be a well-rounded provider you need additional skills to embrace professional practice.

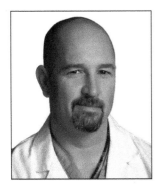

The National Commission for the Certification of Physician Assistants (NCCPA) has now made these skills required and will be up to 5% of the Physician Assistant National Certifying Exam (PANCE.)

We need to learn such areas as professional development, legal/medical ethics, medical informatics, extraordinary patient care and communication, physician/PA relationship and public health.

Professional Practice for Physician Assistant provides clear understandings of the core concepts of the professional practice portion of the PANCE.

Initially, the question seems simple. But, when explored deeper the question becomes critical. The question is, why, in the academic system we have, do we have tests? Well, the initial, simple answer is so we can gauge knowledge. So we know who "knows" and who does not. So, we have tests to have objective proof on knowledge. But, there is a flaw.

We are tested, far too often, in a social system. A social system is manipulative. It's a game. Meaning, if you earn an "A," you must have mastered the content. You are "smart" and are going to be successful. But, we know that isn't really the case. We know, that far too often, the test doesn't really examine knowledge. Most tests evaluate a person's ability to study information in a manner that allows quick recall and then is dumped from the brain. We call it "cramming." It's ineffective, for most people, in true education.

There is a natural system. This is different. You can't cramp. It's like farming and fitness. It's directly proportionate to effort, consistency and effectiveness. There is no "quick fix." All quick diets fail. The only way you are going to get healthy is by the discipline of exercise and saying "no" to foods that feel good but ultimately poison your body. A good test blends academic understanding with worldly expectations. It's the same with the Physician Assistant National Certifying Exam (PANCE.)

In 2019, led by Dawn Morton-Rias, and the National Commission for the Certification of Physician Assistants (NCCPA,) there is an attempt to blend the academic with a clinical practice.

The practice of medicine, as a physician assistant, is much more than antibiotics, pathophysiology of disease and physical exams. Sure, we need foundations; we need building blocks, yet to be a well-rounded provider you need additional skills to embrace professional practice.

The NCCPA has now made these skills required knowledge and will be up to 5% of the PANCE. It's referred to as "professional practice."

We need to learn such areas as professional development, legal/medical ethics, medical informatics, extraordinary patient care and communication, physician/PA relationship and public health.

This book, Professional Practice for Physician Assistant, provides clear understandings of the core concepts of the professional practice portion of the PANCE. But, our hope is that it's more than that. Our hope is this book evolves into a mandatory text that all PAs read to help them thrive.

For anyone who reads this book and finds an area of correction or improvement, please contact us and share your knowledge. We would love that and send you a "thank you" gift. Our expectation is that this book meets the requirements of the NCCPA, but more importantly, becomes a catalyst for your continued growth in your professional practice.

INTRODUCTION

All PA students who graduate from an ARC-PA accredited PA program in the United States take the Physician Assistant National Certifying Examination (PANCE), a multiple-choice, high stakes examination developed by the National Commission on Certification of Physician Assistants (NCCPA). The exam consists of 300 questions divided in to six blocks. In 2018, the NCCPA reported that they were making some changes to the NCCPA PANCE Blueprint, the document that provides PA programs and students information about what will likely be assessed on the PANCE. The changes will be effective in 2019.

While 95% of the exam will still be on medical content and task categories, they are adding a new category called Professional Practice. Professional Practice will be worth 5% of the PANCE. Included in Professional Practice are the following:

• **Legal and medical ethics**

    o Cultural and religious beliefs affecting health care

    o Informed consent, advanced directives, living wills, do not resuscitate, medical power of attorney

    o Common medicolegal issues

    o Patient and provider rights and responsibilities

    o Medical record documentation

• **Medical informatics**

    oBilling and coding

    o Using appropriate medical information sources

• **Patient care and communication**

    o Cultural and religious diversity

    o Health care that is patient specific

    o Patient education regarding end-of-life decisions and informed consent

- **The Physician/PA relationship**

  o Scope of practice

  o Physician supervisory issues

  o Medical malpractice, mandated reporting, conflict of interest, impaired provider

- **Professional development**

  o CME resources

  o Analyzing evidence-based medicine

  o Using epidemiologic techniques

- **Public health and population health**

  o Basic disaster preparedness

  o Infection control measures and response to outbreaks

  o Occupational health issues for healthcare workers and non-healthcare workers

  o Travel health

- **Risk management**

  o Quality improvement, patient safety

This first edition of the Professional Practice Guidebook provides concise and straightforward information about these new topics. We hope that the reader will use this resource to supplement their preparation for the PANCE in 2019. Look for other CME4Life PANCE/PANRE preparation resources at *https://CME4Life.com*

PROFESSIONAL DEVELOPMENT

Continuing medical education[1]

Passing the **PA national certifying exam (the PANCE)** is the first step in what will hopefully be a long and fulfilling career in medicine. The PANCE consists of 300 multiple-choice questions divided in to five blocks of 60 questions. In order to be eligible to take the PANCE, you must have graduated from an Accreditation Review Commission on Education for the PA (ARC-PA) accredited program. Once you have graduated from an ARC-PA accredited PA program, you have six opportunities to pass the PANCE or pass within six years. The NCCPA made modifications to the content areas for the PANCE which will be initiated in 2019. While 95% of the exam still contains questions relating to medical content, up to 20% of exam questions may be general surgery questions and 5% will be professional practice topics.

Exam takers have 60 minutes to complete each block of the PANCE. Once the PA passes the PANCE, they are considered a PA-C, but must still apply for state licensure in each respective state they wish to practice. PAs must still maintain their NCCPA certification by completing 100 hours of continuing medical education (CME) every two years, of which a minimum of 50 must be Category I, plus pass the **Physician Assistant National Recertifying Examination (PANRE)** every 10 years. The traditional PANRE consists of 240 multiple-choice questions divided in to four blocks of 60 questions each. When registering for the PANRE, the PA can choose either adult medicine, primary care, or surgery as a focus area. The focus area will comprise 40% of test questions. Regardless of which focus area is selected, 60% of the PANRE will still consist of primary care questions, and 5% will be Professional Practice questions.

The 2018-2019 alternative to the PANRE pilot program is not a high-stakes, single attempt multiple choice exam. Rather, it consists of 25 questions each quarter for two years. The PA will be provided immediate feedback on right or wrong answers with justification as to why an answer was correct.

The National Commission on the Certification of Physician Assistants (NCCPA)[1] is the organization responsible for administering the certifying and recertifying exams, and it is the responsibility of each PA to log their CME with the NCCPA. The NCCPA charges a fee for maintenance of the certification which must be paid by the end of the year in which the certification will expire. In the past, PAs were required to log 100 hours of CME and pass the recertifying exam every six years. Starting in 2018,

PAs will be able to recertify via the traditional recertifying exam or the new alternative PANRE. Starting in 2014, PAs who were due for recertification were able to enter a 10-year cycle where they must still log 100 hours every two years, but do not have to take a recertifying examination until 10 years.

The new 2019 PANCE:

Medical Categories:	Task areas:
Cardiovascular 13%	Most Likely Diagnosis 18%
Pulmonary 10%	History and Physical Examination 17%
Gastrointestinal/nutrition 9%	Clinical Interventions 14%
Musculoskeletal 8%	Pharmacotherapeutics 14%
ENT 7%	Diagnostic and Laboratory Studies 12%
Endocrine 7%	Prevention, Patient Education, and Health Maintenance 10%
Neurologic 7%	Basic Science 10%
Reproductive 7%	*Professional Practice 5%
Infectious disease 6%	
Behavioral medicine 6%	
Dermatology 5%	
Renal 5%	
Hematology 5%	
Genitourinary (male and female) 5%	

Professional Practice items are what this book is based upon.

Category I CME is educational experiences that have been peer-reviewed and vetted to ensure they meet strict criteria set by CME accreditors, such as the American Academy of Physician Assistants (AAPA), the American Medical Association, the American Osteopathic Association, the American Council for Continuing Medical Education, or the American Academy of Family Physicians. Specific certifications and credentials can qualify for Category I CME, including Advanced Cardiac Life Support and Pediatric Advanced Life Support, both offered through the American Heart Association. Another option for Category I CME is Performance Improvement CME, or PI-CME. Performance Improvement utilizes a systematic approach to clinical quality improvements. While no longer required, the NCCPA will double the first 20 credits of PI-CME for each logging cycle. Self-assessment CME utilizes a systematic approach to an individual's knowledge, performance, or skills and builds on ways to improve knowledge, performance, or skills. The NCCPA currently affords a multiplier of 1.5 for every credit of Self-Assessment CME that is completed.

Category II CME is a medical educational activity that does not meet Category I requirements, but still can provide opportunities for PAs to expand their knowledge about medicine, patient care, and the role of the PA. Industry-sponsored events are typically considered Category 2 events.

In addition to maintaining PA certification, PAs can choose to seek a **Certificate of Added Qualifications (CAQ)**. To apply for a CAQ certificate, the PA must be currently certified as a PA-C and have an unrestricted state or territory license (or demonstrate unrestricted privileges in a U.S. government agency). In addition, the PA must complete a minimum of 150 hours of Category I CME in their chosen specialty, of which at least 50 must have been completed within the two years before applying for the CAQ; have at least one year (a minimum of 2000 hours) of clinical experience in that specialty; provide physician verification of the PA's specialty practice; and successful passing of the specialty exam. Successful CAQ certification remains valid for 10 years. Current areas of specialty practice are cardiovascular and thoracic surgery, orthopedic surgery, emergency medicine, hospital medicine, nephrology, pediatrics, and psychiatry.

Reference:

1. Maintaining certification. National Commission on the Certification of Physician Assistants. nccpa.net. https://www.nccpa.net/CertificationProcess. Accessed on 5/11/2018.

For more information:

http://prodcmsstoragesa.blob.core.windows.net/uploads/files/PANCEBlueprint.pdf

PATIENT CARE AND COMMUNICATION
(individual patients)

Affordable and effective health care that is patient specific

Patient-centered care is medical care that is "respectful of, and responsive to, individual patient preferences, needs, and values," and that care decisions are made with consideration of individual patient values and needs[1]. The Institute of Medicine (IOM), now called the National Academy of Medicine (NAM), also outlines several aspects of patient-centered care that includes integration and coordination of health care; appropriate and adequate information regarding all aspects of care, including diagnoses and prognoses; physical comfort; emotional support; involving patients' friends and family in the care of patients; and access to and continuity of care. All of these aspects require PAs to have an understanding of the cultural, social, economic, and emotional needs and wants of their patients. Integrating patient-centered care also requires PAs to provide a balance between evidence-based medicine and the patients' individual wants and needs.

The experiences of patients correlate with health outcomes.[2] Patients who report more positive interactions with their health care provider tend to have better outcomes. Providers who receive positive marks on patient surveys have lower malpractice claims. On a Likert scale of five steps, from very poor to very good, each negative drop in a score correlated with a 21% risk of being named in a malpractice suit. [3]The strongest predictor of a positive rating by a patient is the patient's perception of the communication with their provider(s), and patients who perceive to have positive communication with their provider report stronger adherence to provider recommendations regarding their care.[3,4,5]

Beginning in October 2012, the Hospital Consumer Assessment of Healthcare Providers and Systems (HCAHPS) survey has been used to track patient satisfaction. The HCAHPS survey was developed by the Agency for Healthcare Research and Quality (AHRQ). The Center for Medicare and Medicaid Services (CMS) offers financial incentives to hospitals and hospital systems that is based upon quality measures, including the results of HCAHPS surveys. The vendor Press Ganey Associates is an authorized distributor of the HCAHPS survey.[6]

The Centers for Medicare and Medicaid Services has used surveys to help track quality of care indicators. Health plans that participate in Medicare and Medicaid service provision are required to administer the HCAHPS Health Plan Survey as part of their accreditation. Health plans must not only report on patient satisfaction and outcomes, but on processes for improvement.[6]

Press Ganey Associates has supplied patient satisfaction surveys to hospitals and hospital systems for many years, but their data collection and analysis has been widely criticized[7]. For example, a minimum of 30 survey responses in a specified period of time is required to provide data that would be statistically significant, but Press Ganey Associates have been known to collect data on much smaller sample sizes and report results. In addition, critics of the patient satisfaction surveys have pointed out that there are many other variables that can affect a patient's perception of how well a provider or hospital met their needs. Retrospective analyses of the relationship between patient satisfaction scores and inpatient utilization reveal that patients perceive a higher level of satisfaction when utilization of services increases, but does not correlate with decreased morbidity rates. Another criticism is that patient satisfaction can vary depending on their cultural, racial, and even geographic orientation.[8]

Use of patient satisfaction surveys can identify areas for improvement and have been implemented among many healthcare providers and plans as part of their formal quality improvement programs. The data collected can help not only identify areas of improvement, but provide information about what is being done well and what has improved, but care must be taken to not make inappropriate inferences when there are small sample sizes or other external variables that can affect data analysis.

References:

1. Institute of Medicine. 2001.
http://www.nationalacademies.org/hmd/~/media/Files/Report%20Files/2001/Crossing-the-Quality-Chasm/Quality%20Chasm%202001%20%20report%20brief.pdf

2. Sequist TD, Schneider EC, Anastario M, et al. Quality monitoring of physicians: linking patients' experiences of care to clinical quality and outcomes. *J Gen Intern Med* 2008; 23(11):1784-90.

3. Fullam F, Garman AN, Johnson TJ, et al. The use of patient satisfaction surveys and alternate coding procedures to predict malpractice risk. *Med Care 2009* May; 47(5):1-7

4. Levinson W, Roter DL, Mullooly JP, et al. Physician-patient communication: the relationship with malpractice claims among primary care physicians and surgeons. *JAMA* 1997; 277:553-9.

5.   Zolnierek KB, Dimatteo MR. Physician communication and patient adherence to treatment: a meta-analysis. *Med Care* 2009; 47(3): 213-20

6.   About CAHPS. The Agency for Healthcare Research and Quality. 2018. https://www.ahrq.gov/cahps/about-cahps/index.html

7.   Sullivan W, DeLucia J. 2+2=7? Seven things you may not know about Press Ganey Statistics. *Emergency Physicians Monthly*. September 22, 2010. Available at: http://www.epmonthly.com/archives/ features/227-seven-things-you-may-not-know-aboutpress-gainey-statistics/.

8.   Zusman EE. HCAHPS Replaces Press Ganey Survey as Quality Measure for Patient Hospital Experience. August 2012. *Neurosurgery.* 71(2).

REDUCING HEALTHCARE DISPARITIES

Healthcare disparities are differences in the health and healthcare between people from various populations. The differences are socially determined[1], cannot be explained by patient needs and preferences or treatment recommendations, and are considered unjust. The terms health inequalities and health inequities are used interchangeably. Populations that experience healthcare disparities can be ethnic or racial, socioeconomic, geographic, sexual oriented, and/or gender-based. Other barriers to quality healthcare include education, safety, language, culture, provider bias, finances, and delivery systems. Disparities not only affect the people who experience barriers to care but create a significant financial strain on the healthcare system. Thus, healthcare disparities affect us all.

Over 50% of the population in the U.S. is projected to be people of color by 2045.[1] People of color and low-income people experience significant barriers to care and have worse outcomes. In addition, they are more likely to be uninsured.[2]

Blacks, Alaska Natives, and American Indians have a higher prevalence of certain chronic diseases, such as diabetes, cardiovascular disease, and asthma than Non-Hispanic Whites.[2] The disparity among HIV and AIDS diagnoses is most apparent in that the incidence among Blacks is ten times higher than Whites.[3] In addition, infant mortality rates are still higher among Black women compared to Whites, as are maternal morbidity and mortality.[3]

Healthcare disparities also affect people who are gay, lesbian, bisexual, and transgender.[4] Bias and access issues present challenges to members of this population. Adolescents who are gay, bisexual, or experiencing gender identity conflict are more likely to be homeless, lack health insurance, use illicit drugs and alcohol, or have depression and anxiety.[4,5]

Patients who are confined to their homes due to mobility issues, live alone, have few social contacts, have no reliable means of transportation, or have home security issues are more likely to die during a heat wave.[6] People with less formal education are more likely to die from all-cause mortality than people with advanced education. Multiple studies over time have shown that there is a social gradient within the U.S. where people of lower socioeconomic status have worse outcomes and less quality of life indicators than people of higher socioeconomic status. Some researchers have proposed that one reason we see such disparities along socioeconomic status grades is due to chronic stress, the type of chronic stress where one does not feel safe in their environment, has little social support, or little social status. Others purport that if someone feels as if life is out of their control, they will be more likely to suffer from poor health. Thus, economic inequality is a major driver of health disparities in the U.S.

The Centers for Medicare and Medicaid Services developed an Accountable Health Communities Model that helps to identify and mitigate the social needs that affect health of Medicare and Medicaid beneficiaries.[7] The work of the Model is accomplished through an integrated process of identification and referral to appropriate agencies and community resources. There are slightly over 30 organizations, mostly in the northeastern U.S., participating in the Model. Some areas that have been identified as having a negative effect on the health of participants include poor housing, food insecurity, and interpersonal violence.

A 2009 study[8] revealed that the elimination of minority health disparities would have lowered direct medical expenses by $229.4 billion and indirect medical expenses by over $one trillion between 2003 – 2006. Indirect costs include lost work wages due to disability or illness and premature death.

Increasing patients' health literacy can reduce some of the disparities in the U.S. Patients with low health literacy are more likely to be elderly, immigrants, rural, socioeconomically disadvantaged, and be of a minority group.[9] Many of these patients do not understand written materials given to them regarding their health and their provider visits, and they struggle to understand basic health information.

Ways to mitigate health disparities include:

• Increasing access to primary care services through strengthening payments and providing financial incentives to healthcare providers who work in underserved areas.

• Reducing the barriers to insurance, including issues regarding co-pays and deductibles.

• Defining and integrating value-based care over volume when paying healthcare providers.

• Continuing to research healthcare disparities, looking at what is working and what needs improvement.

• Reducing bias in medicine.

• Increasing racial and ethnic diversity in our profession.

• Providing culturally appropriate care to all patients.

References:

1. "Social Determinants of Health: Definitions," Centers for Disease Control and Prevention, accessed published March 2014, http://www.cdc.gov/socialdeterminants/Definitions.html.

2.   Agency for Healthcare Research and Quality, *Agency for Healthcare Research and Quality: Division of Priority Populations*, (Rockville, MD: Agency for Healthcare Research and Quality, April 2016), http://www.ahrq.gov/sites/default/files/wysiwyg/research/findings/factsheets/priority-populations/prioritypopulations_factsheet.pdf.

3. The Kaiser Family Foundation State Health Facts. Data Source: Census Bureau's March 2015 Current Population Survey, "Poverty Rate by Race/Ethnicity. (2014)," accessed July 20, 2016, http://www.statehealthfacts.org/comparemaptable.jsp?ind=14&cat=1&sub=2&yr=274&typ=2.

4. Kaiser Family Foundation, *Key Facts on Health and Health Care by Race and Ethnicity*, (Washington, DC: Kaiser Family Foundation, June 2016), http://files.kff.org/attachment/Chartpack-Key-Facts-on-Health-and-Health-Care-by-Race-and-Ethnicity.

5. Kaiser Family Foundation, *Health And Access to Care and Coverage for Lesbian, Gay, Bisexual, and Transgender Individuals in the U.S.*, (Washington, DC: Kaiser Family Foundation, June 2016), http://kff.org/disparities-policy/issue-brief/health-and-access-to-care-and-coverage-for-lesbian-gay-bisexual-and-transgender-individuals-in-the-u-s/.

6. Barr DA. The relationship between socioeconomic status and health, or, "They call it 'poor health' for a reason." In Barr DA. *Health Disparities in the United States: Social Class, Race, Ethnicity, and Health.* Baltimore: The Johns Hopkins University Press; 2008.

7. Accountable Health Communities Model," Centers for Medicare & Medicaid Services, revised May 18, 2016, https://innovation.cms.gov/initiatives/AHCM.

8. Thomas LaVeist, Darrell Gaskin, and Patrick Richard, *The Economic Burden of Health Inequalities in the United States*, (Washington, DC: Joint Center for Political and Economic Studies, September 2009), http://www.hhnmag.com/ext/resources/inc-hhn/pdfs/resources/Burden_Of_Health_FINAL_0.pdf.

9.   Abercrombie DD. Chapter 39: Health disparities. In Ballweg R, et al. *Physician Assistant: A Guide to Clinical Practice.* 5th ed. Philadelphia, PA: Elsevier; 2013.

For more information:

Kaiser Family Foundation, *Key Facts on Health and Health Care by Race and Ethnicity,* (Washington, DC: Kaiser Family Foundation, June 2016), http://files.kff.org/attachment/Chartpack-Key-Facts-on-Health-and-Health-Care-by-Race-and-Ethnicity.

Paula Braverman et al., "Socioeconomic Disparities in Health in the United States: What the Patterns Tell Us," *American Journal of Public Health* 100(1) (April 2010):186-196.

U.S. Department of Health and Human Services, *HHS Action Plan to Reduce Racial and Ethnic Disparities: Implementation Progress Report 2011-2014,* (Washington, DC: U.S. Department of Health and Human Services, November 2015), http://minorityhealth.hhs.gov/assets/pdf/FINAL_HHS_Action_Plan_Progress_Report_11_2_2015.pdf.

CULTURAL COMPETENCY

Cultural and religious beliefs related to health care

Culture is defined as a system of values, beliefs, and customs that a group of people use to navigate through social experiences. Often, people in a cultural group will share a language, a religion, a dress code, and even food preferences. The way in which **people define and experience health and illness is largely related to one's cultural orientation**. Thus, an individual's cultural identity will directly influence the care of the patient, so it is important for the health care provider to be aware of their patients' cultural orientation and their own potential biases.

Each encounter with a patient can be considered a cultural exchange.[1] It is our responsibility as PAs to avail ourselves of information regarding the beliefs and practices of the people we serve if we are to be effective care givers. However, there is a danger in overgeneralizing the beliefs and practices of a cultural or ethnic group, as subcultures exist within these groups, and beliefs and practices can be affected by level of education, acculturation, and socioeconomic status.[1] The IOM, now called the National Academy of Medicine, maintains that health care providers should offer **patient-centered care** that employs appropriate communication to improve the quality of health care provided and eliminate cultural and ethnic disparities.

Some examples of the disparities that have been documented in the U.S. include the following:

• Non-Hispanic whites were more likely to be referred for cardiac catheterization than African Americans/Blacks[2] and have overall better cardiovascular event outcomes than all other ethnic groups.[3]

• Non-Hispanic whites were more likely to receive pain medication in the emergency department for long-bone fractures than Hispanics.[4]

• European Americans are about 25% less likely to develop end-stage renal disease than African Americans/Blacks, and when on dialysis, African Americans/Blacks are significantly less likely to be referred for transplantation.[5,6]

• African Americans/Blacks with dyslipidemia are less likely to be taking statin drugs.[7]

• Non-Hispanic blacks, Hispanics, and non-Hispanic Asians have lower immunization rates than non-Hispanic whites.[8]

• Hispanics and Asians had higher rates of hospital-acquired infections than non-Hispanic whites.[9]

Differences among and between various groups exist. Immigration status, language, and length of time in the US all affect how individuals from different groups navigate healthcare in the U.S. While it is dangerous to assume knowledge of the beliefs and practices about non-Hispanic whites, what follows are some thoughts to ponder about the patients we serve.

The Asian Population

The United States Census Bureau lists twenty Asian groups based on origin. They include Chinese, Filipino, Indian, Vietnamese, Korean, Japanese, Pakistani, Burmese Pakistani, Cambodian, Hmong, Thai, Laotian, Bangladeshi, Burmese, Indonesian, Nepalese, Sri Lankan, Malaysian, Bhutanese, Mongolian, and Okinowan.[10]. The six largest groups in the United States are Chinese, Filipino, Indian, Vietnamese, Korean, and Japanese.[10] Health care workers are likely to encounter Asians from all twenty nations of origin with very distinct beliefs and practices. The Chinese who adhere to traditional beliefs may think of health as being in physical and spiritual harmony with nature, a belief deeply rooted in Taoism.[11] However, not all Asians are Taoists. Some are Christian, Buddhist, Hindu, and Confucianist, so it is helpful for the health care provider to ask about a patient's religious beliefs, particularly when discussing chronic illness and end-of-life care.

Many Asians and non-Asians will utilize Chinese medical practices, including acupuncture and herbs, to treat illness. Acupuncture has been used for thousands of years, and there is an evidence-based body of literature to support its utility. The most common tradition health belief system in Asia is ayurveda. Ayurveda uses thousands of herbal preparations. There are many resources available to help guide discussions about traditional herbal products for medicinal purposes. For example, a PubMed search with the keywords Chinese+herbal+medicine+systematic+review retrieved over 3000 evidence-based articles on a myriad of medical topics, including hypertension, depression, gout, and even COPD. For a quick review of common herbal products, visit the webpage https://nccih.nih.gov/health/herbsataglance.htm.

The Native American/Alaska Eskimo Population

There are 562 federally recognized Native American nations in the United States, with the majority residing in Alaska.[12] They are ethnically, culturally, and linguistically diverse, but do share some common themes. These themes are deep in the historical narrative of the Native American and Alaska Eskimo populations and demand respect. For example, American Indians generally do not believe in the germ theory of disease; rather, illness is "the price to pay" for events that may have already occurred or will occur in the future.[11] Illness may also be caused by evil spirits, breaking a taboo, misusing sacred rituals, and even attempting to contact witches.

Some Native Americans may have a deep distrust of the American health system. Often this is due to disagreements between the patient and the health care provider regarding the etiology and treatment of disease. Native Americans may use herbs and other complementary techniques to treat illness and maintain health. When caring for a Native American patient, PAs must ask questions respectfully and listen carefully, but taking notes during the interview is considered offensive.[11]

The African American/Black Population

As mentioned above, African Americans/Blacks generally have worse outcomes in certain diseases, such as cancer and cardiovascular care. Maternal morbidity and mortality rates are worse for African American/Black women than all other racial/ethnic groups.[13] While caring for any patient, it is important not to assume lifestyles, beliefs, or cultural identity. Again, ask respectful questions and be willing to listen. Like other ethnic and cultural minority groups, access to health care is often a problem. There is a deep distrust of the American health system, due in part to the debacle of the syphilis experiments in Macon County, Alabama during the late 1930s into the 1940s[14] and the misuse of Henrietta Lack's cells.[15] Many African American/Black patients may also feel as though their providers "talk down" to them and feel the insidious racism evident in many communities. As PAs, we need to acknowledge and recognize these feelings, and begin to understand the perspectives of each our patients as individuals and as members of our communities.

The Hispanic Population

In the United States, the majority of Hispanic patients are from Mexico.[16] Many Hispanic patients are undocumented. The fear of being identified as living illegally in the United States is often a reason many Hispanic patients avoid seeking medical care until it is too late. For some, taking time off work and the loss of wages associated with time off from work is too burdensome. Also, many are non-English speakers and there can be significant language barriers.[11] If a PA is taking care of a Hispanic patient, and the patient has presented late in the disease, it is important to recognize some of these barriers to care and avoid harsh judgment of the patient.

Like many of our patients, Hispanic patients may have deep spiritual beliefs.[11] Often, they will bring several family members in to the clinic with them to provide emotional support. If the patient does not speak English, it is inappropriate to have family members translate. In addition, some patients will use traditional herbs and teas to treat illness. Always ask about any non-pharmaceutical supplement the patient may be using.

Religious Issues

Patients' **religious and spiritual beliefs** can affect the provision of health care as well as a patient's understanding about quality of life. End-of-life discussions must consider a patient's religious beliefs.[18] Jehovah's Witness patients may refuse blood products on the basis of their religious beliefs. Some deeply religious patients may choose not to undergo chemotherapy, radiation therapy, or other life-prolonging therapies because they embrace death as a way to heaven. Religious beliefs can affect a patient's perspective on pregnancy, particularly if an anomaly is discovered. While we do not have to agree with the beliefs of our patients, we must always respect those beliefs unless a minor's health is at risk.

Conclusion

Helping take care of patients from different backgrounds is not only inevitable in the United States but can be a tremendous source of joy and discovery. People from different ethnic, cultural, and religious groups sometimes share beliefs and traditions, but it is important for the PA not to assume anything about any patient. Overgeneralization can be dangerous as it may negatively affect care. Always listen and learn from the patient, and **when a patient does not speak English, you must offer language assistance from a properly trained individual.**

Cultural competency is a process. Cultural humility can be integrated into the ongoing process of becoming more culturally competent. Cultural humility requires the PA to be open to a patient's cultural identity, particularly aspects of their identity that they have identified as being most important. It is also important to develop a commitment to self-reflection and a desire to help repair societal power imbalances by advocating for others who may lack power[19].

The US Department of Health and Human Services offers online training in cultural and language appropriate care. Completion of the training provides nine hours of continuing medical education and can be found at https://www.thinkculturalhealth.hhs.gov/education/physicians.

References:

1. Fortin, A.H., Dwamena, F.C., Frankel, R.M., and Smith, R.C. (2012). *Smith's patient-centered interviewing: An evidence-based method, 3rd edition.* New York: McGraw Hill Medical

2. Chen J, Rathore SS, Radford MJ, Wang Y, Krumholz HM . Racial differences in the use of cardiac catheterization after acute myocardial infarction. *N Engl J Med.* 2001 May;344(19):1443-9.

3. Ski CF, King-Shier KM, Thomson DR. Gender, socioeconomic and ethnic/racial disparities in cardiovascular disease: a time for change. *Int J Cardiol.* 2014 Jan 1;170(3):255-7. doi: 10.1016/j.ijcard.2013.10.082. Epub 2013 Nov 1.

4. Todd KH, Samaroo N, Hoffman JR. Ethnicity as a risk factor for inadequate emergency department analgesia. *JAMA.* 1993;269(12):1537

5. Epstein AM, Ayanian JZ, Keogh JH, Noonan SJ, Armistead N, Cleary PD, Weissman JS, David-Kasdan JA, Carlson D, Fuller J, Marsh D, Conti RM. Racial disparities in access to renal transplantation--clinically appropriate or due to underuse or overuse? *N Engl J Med.* 2000;343(21):1537.

6. Ayanian JZ, Cleary PD, Weissman JS, Epstein AM. The effect of patients' preferences on racial differences in access to renal transplantation. *N Engl J Med.* 1999;341(22):1661.

7. Clark LT, Maki KC, Galant R, Maron DJ, Pearson TA, Davidson MH. Ethnic differences in achievement of cholesterol treatment goals. Results from the National Cholesterol Education Program Evaluation Project Utilizing Novel E-Technology II. *J Gen Intern Med.* 2006;21(4):320.

8. Lu P, O'Halloran AO, Williams WW, Lindley MC, Farrall S, Bridges CB. Racial and Ethnic Disparities in Vaccination Coverage Among Adult Populations in the U.S. *Am J Prev Med.* 2015 Dec; 49(6 Suppl 4):S412-S425. doi: 10.1016/ j.amepre. 2015.03.005

9. Bakullari A, Metersky ML, Wang Y, Eldridge N, Eckenrode S, Pandolfi MM, Jaser L, Galusha D, Moy E. Racial and ethnic disparities in healthcare-associated infections in the United States, 2009-2011. *Infect Control Hosp Epidemiol.* 2014 Oct;35 Suppl 3:S10-6. doi: 10.1086/677827.

10. Pew Research. (4 April 2014). *Asian American demographics.* Retrieved from http://www.pewsocialtrends.org/2013/04/04/asian-groups-in-the-u-s/

11. Spector, R.E. (2013). Cultural diversity in health and illness, 8th edition. Needham, MA: Pearson

12. National Congress of American Indians. (n.d.). An introduction to Indian nations in the United States. Retrieved from http://www.ncai.org/about-tribes/indians_101.pdf

13. Howell EA, Zeitlin J, Hebert P, Balbierz A, Egorova N. Paradoxical trends and racial differences in obstetric quality and neonatal and maternal mortality. *Obstet Gynecol.* 2013 Jun;121(6):1201-8. doi: 10.1097/AOG.0b013e3182932238.

14. Tuskegee University. (n.d.). *About the USPHS syphilis study.* Retrieved fromhttp://www.tuskegee.edu/about_us/centers_of_excellence/bioethics_center/about_ the_usphs_syphilis_study.aspx

15. Samuel L. 5 ways Henrietta Lacks changed medical science. Scientific American, April 2017. https://www.scientificamerican.com/article/5-ways-henrietta-lacks-changed-medical-science/

16. Flores, A. How the US Hispanic population is changing. Sept 18, 2017. Pew Research Center. http://www.pewresearch.org/fact-tank/2017/09/18/how-the-u-s-hispanic-population-is-changing/

17. United States Department of Health and Human Services. (n.d.). *Think cultural health.* Retrieved from https://www.thinkculturalhealth.hhs.gov/content /clas.asp

18. Ellison CJ & Benjamins MR. Invited Commentary. Provision of spiritual support to patients with advanced cancer by religious communities and associations with medical care at the end of life. JAMA Intern Med. 2013;173(12):1117-1118. doi:10.1001/jamainternmed.2013.922

19. American Psychological Association. Reflections on cultural humility. 2013. apa.org. http://www.apa.org/pi/families/resources/newsletter/2013/08/cultural-humility.aspx. Accessed on June 26, 2018.

Further reading:

US Department of Health and Human Services. https://www.thinkculturalhealth.hhs.gov/clas/standards

QUALITY IMPROVEMENT AND RISK MANAGEMENT

Medical errors are responsible for thousands of deaths every year in the United States.[1] According to the Centers for Disease Control and Prevention (CDC), **medical errors would rate sixth as a leading cause of death in the U.S.** Not only do medical errors cost lives and cause unnecessary morbidity, it costs the healthcare system and society billions of dollars annually. The National Quality Forum and the Joint Commission have listed several events that should never occur and if they do, an immediate investigation is undertaken. Called sentinel events, these are events that negatively effects a patient and can result in death, permanent disability or harm, or severe temporary harm that requires interventions to sustain life.[1]

Some of the sentinel events include:[2]

• Discharge of newborn to the wrong family.

• Unanticipated death of a newborn.

• Surgery performed on the wrong person or the wrong body part.

• Radiation therapy given to the wrong person or the wrong body part.

• Surgical instruments and objects left in a body cavity.

• Severe neonatal jaundice (bilirubin >30 mg/dL).

• Rape within a facility.

• Suicide within a facility or within 72 hours after discharge.

• Transfusion reaction due to blood group incompatibility.

• Assault of a patient.

• Abduction of a patient.

• Pressure ulcers that are stage 3 or 4 after the patient was admitted.

• Medication errors.

Medication errors are common. They can occur anywhere during the time the prescription is written or transmitted and when the patient receives the medication. Adverse drug effects are not always due to medication errors. The Joint Commission considers reducing medication errors a national priority.[3]

A landmark in the quality movement in health care was the publication of the IOM (now called the National Academy of Medicine) report "To Err is Human: Building a Safer Health System" in 1999. Medical risk management focuses on risk reduction through improvement of patient care, but a criticism of medical risk management is that it is reactive, retrospective, and at times, punitive.[2]

Medical risk management is a three-step process:

- identifying risk;

- avoiding or minimizing the risk of loss; and

- reducing the impact of losses when they occur.

Within medical risk management, safety and quality are closely related, **but risk managers tend to focus on limiting liability of the organization and reducing future risk.** Thus, risk managers may be strongly oriented towards financial loss through medical malpractice claims.

Quality improvement (QI), on the other hand, engages in prospective and retrospective reviews. At its core, **quality improvement is aimed at overall healthcare improvement** from a systems perspective and a patient care perspective to improve patient care quality. This process involves measuring what you are doing now and creating ways to do things better. Patient experiences and patient satisfaction have become part of the accepted quality indicators of care.[4]

Where medical risk management tends to attribute blame, quality improvement aims to avoid blame by creating systems that prevent errors from occurring. QI specifically attempts to avoid attributing blame, and to create systems to prevent errors from happening.

The American Academy of Family Physicians (AAFP) provides information on quality measures in their practice management section of their website.[5]

Some of their recommendations include:

• A **"culture of quality"** should be established in the practice. This includes actions and attitudes that reflect and support the commitment to quality improvement.

• Develop **dedicated teams** to identify areas that could be improved. Some of these areas could be delays in care, low worker morale, high-risk patient populations, and communication barriers.

• **Data** should be collected and analyzed throughout the quality improvement process, beginning with baseline data before any quality improvement efforts are initiated, and then again at the end. It is important to track changes over time. Please see discussion below about how to develop quality measures.

• Openly **communicate** quality improvement activities and results to all stakeholders, including healthcare providers, staff, and even patients.

• If the practice wraps up a quality improvement effort and the results show that the improvement worked, do not stop there. **Continue to search** out new ways to improve the practice. Talk to patients, staff, and healthcare providers and solicit their input.

• Finally, do not be afraid to **share** with others.

How does one develop an appropriate metric? The AAFP[5] and the National Quality Forum provide guidance on developing a quality measure. These include:

• The **importance** of the metric. Is it evidence-based? Does it occur frequently enough to justify a quality improvement project? What impact will it have on patient outcomes?

• The **measurability** of the metric. Is it even measurable? Will the results be reliable and valid?

• The **achievability** of the metric. Is it even possible to capture the data?

• The **usefulness** of the metric and subsequent data. Once data is collected, can the information be used in a meaningful way?

• The ability of the metrics to be **aligned**. The Centers for Medicaid and Medicare Services (CMS) developed a Core Quality Measures Collaborative that provides specific information on metrics that have been used in other successful quality improvement efforts.[6]

o They are divided into the following categories, and can be found here: https://www.cms.gov/Medicare/Quality-Initiatives-Patient-Assessment-Instruments/QualityMeasures/index.html

• Primary care, patient centered medical homes, and accountable care organizations.

• Cardiology

• Gastroenterology

• Hepatitis C and HIV

• Medical oncology

• Obstetrics and gynecology

• Pediatrics

• Orthopedics

Resources to help develop appropriate metrics include: Agency for Healthcare Research and Quality (www.qualitymeasures.ahrq.gov), National Quality Forum (www.qualityforum.org), and the Quality Payment Program(qpp.cms.gov).

In 2015, the Medicare Access and CHIP Reauthorization Act (MACRA) was signed into law.[7] This piece of legislation modifies how PAs and other healthcare providers receive rewards for implementing changes in their practices that would improve the quality of care rendered to Medicare and Medicaid recipients. The new Merit Based Incentive Payments System (MIPS) combines several quality-oriented federal programs under one umbrella. There are four performance measures: quality, advancing care information (formerly known as Meaningful Use), improvement activities, and cost. PAs can participate in MIPS if certain practice criteria are met. If the practice sees more than 200 Medicare beneficiaries, bills over $90,000 for Medicare Part B services, and does not participate in a federally sponsored alternative payment model, the PAs, NPs, and physicians in that practice can participate.[7]

The CMS establishes **National Patient Safety Goals** that are updated annually. Maintenance of accreditation demands that healthcare facilities meet or exceed these goals. PAs can identify areas where quality improvement efforts can improve patient care above and beyond the goals of CMS. The AAPA and the NCCPA recognize the importance of quality improvement efforts. PAs who engage in Category I (PI-CME will be granted a doubling of the first 20 credits of the PI-CME per CME logging cycle. For more information about CME, see the section on Professional Development: continuing medical education.

References:

1. The Joint Commission. Sentinel events policies and procedures. June 29, 2017. https://www.jointcommission.org/sentinel_event_policy_and_procedures/. Accessed on June 26, 2018.

2. Cobb TG. Chapter 40: Patient safety and quality of care. In Ballweg R, et al. *Physician Assistant: A Guide to Clinical Practice.* 5th ed. Philadelphia, PA: Elsevier; 2013

3. Agency for Healthcare Research and Quality. Medication errors. ahrq.gov. June 2017. https://psnet.ahrq.gov/primers/primer/23/medication-errors. Accessed on June 26, 2018.

4. United States Department of Health and Human Services, Health Resources and Services Administration. (2011). Quality Improvement. https://www.hrsa.gov/sites/default/files/quality/toolbox/508pdfs/qualityimprovement.pdf

5. Quality measures. American Academy of Family Physicians. 2018. https://www.aafp.org/practice-management/improvement/measures.html. 2018. Accessed on 5/25/2018.

6. Core measures. Centers for Medicaid and Medicare Services. cms.gov. 2017. www.cms.gov/Medicare-Initiatives-Patient-Assessment-Instruments/QualityMeasures/Core-Measures.html

7. Centers for Medicaid And Medicare Services. MIPS overview. https://qpp.cms.gov/mips/overview. Accessed on June 26, 2018.

LEGAL ISSUES AND MEDICAL ETHICS

Introduction to medical ethical concepts[1]

PAs are medical professionals, trained to diagnose and treat patients throughout their lifespan. A professional, by definition, is someone who has undergone specialized advanced training, provides a service to society, embodies intellectualism, and undergoes rigorous certification requirements. Professionalism in medicine requires the PA to act in the patient's best interest, work within their scope of practice, and utilize good judgment regarding patients and the health systems in which they care for patients.

Professionalism also requires the PA to maintain professional growth through required continued medical education that enhances and builds upon medical knowledge and skills and engage in a continuous self-reflective process that allows the PA to further develop the attitudes, character, and virtue of a highly skilled professional.

The common ethical theories used in the U.S. include:

• *Utilitarianism:* we should do what provides the greatest good for the greatest number of people.

• *Deontology:* we have a duty to adhere to rules, i.e. the Ten Commandments.

• *Virtue:* we should act out of courage, justice, charity, and wisdom.

• *Feminist:* based upon the principle of equal rights for men and women, because we value our personal relationships, we should act on behalf of our patients whom we care about.

• *Principlism:* we should act out of a prima facie duty that is obligatory based upon the principles of beneficence, justice, and non-injury.

The common principles that underlie medical ethics in the US include:

• *Autonomy:* freedom of choice, self-determination, and privacy. Patients have a right to choose treatments or behaviors so long as they do not intentionally inflict harm on others.

• *Nonmaleficence:* we should not inflict harm on others. However, we must balance harms with benefits. Cardiac surgery is not without risk (or potential harm), but do the benefits outweigh the risks?

• *Beneficence:* we should work to prevent harm to our patients. We must act in the best interest of the patient. This can sometimes conflict with the concept of paternalism, where we act out of an implied authority that restricts patient freedom.

• *Justice:* we ought to treat people fairly and equitably. But what if resources are scarce? Who gets to have life-saving surgery or medications?

Professionalism requires us to act with integrity, honesty, and respect for the patients we serve. By being mindful of ethical principles, we can begin to work through potentially difficult clinical scenarios with clarity and advocate for our patients' well-being.

Reference:

1. Gianola FJ, Wick KH. Chapter 35: Clinical Ethics. In Ballweg R, et al. *Physician Assistant: A Guide to Clinical Practice.* 5th ed. Philadelphia, PA: Elsevier; 2013.

MANDATED REPORTING [1,2]

PAs are mandated reporters, meaning that it is an ethical and professional responsibility to report any suspected abuse of children, elders, domestic partners/spouses, and other vulnerable populations. Most U.S. jurisdictions require reporting if you have a reasonable suspicion or a reasonable cause to believe that abuse of another has occurred. It is not the responsibility of the PA to investigate. Which agency to report to can vary, so be familiar with whom to contact when abuse is suspected. Remember also that sexual abuse is considered a criminal offense in most jurisdictions, so the local police should be notified.

If child abuse is suspected, the parents or caregivers of the child should be made aware that a report is being filed. Avoid asking questions that would seem interrogative. Begin by summarizing the findings in a non-accusatory or threatening tone.

Some suggestions include:

"The physical examination shows concerning findings, so we have to report to XYZ to make sure the child is safe."

"The physical examination shows unexpected findings given the history, so we need to file a report with XYZ to investigate."

In all cases of suspected abuse, documentation of the history and physical examination must be clear and concise, but provide as many details as possible. Identify the historian and others present in the room. Use the historian's own words in quotes when appropriate. It is advisable to avoid using medical abbreviations. Take photographs of physical abnormalities but include a narrative about each abnormality that is found. In the plan, clearly state why there is a suspicion of abuse using plain language that a non-medical person could easily understand.

Be familiar with the statutes that apply and the agencies that must be contacted if any abuse is suspected. Consequences to failure to report suspected abuse include monetary fines, incarceration, and/or revocation or suspension of the medical license.

Human trafficking is a major problem in the U.S. Adults, adolescents, and children from the U.S. are trafficked into the sex industry and in forced labor. Sometimes people are brought to the U.S. as foreign nationals to work illegally in the sex and labor industry. Human trafficking is modern slavery and traffickers face federal prosecution if caught.

Some signs that a person is being trafficked include:[3]

- Unable to come and go from place to place.

- Is a minor and is performing commercial sex acts.

- Has a pimp.

- Works long hours without breaks and has unusual restrictions while at work.

- Lives in housing that prohibits free entry and exit.

- Exhibits signs of post-traumatic stress disorder, anxiety, depression, trauma.

- Appears malnourished.

- May have tattoo brandings on their body.

- Few or no personal possessions, including an identification.

- Is accompanied by someone else who speaks for the patient.

As with child abuse, the role of the PA is not to investigate. Report suspicions of human trafficking to the National Human Trafficking Hotline: 888-373-7888; text HELP to: 233733; or go on the website: https://humantraffickinghotline.org

References:

1. Child Welfare Information Gateway. (2016). Penalties for failure to report and false reporting of child abuse and neglect. Washington, DC: U.S. Department of Health and Human Services, Children's Bureau.

2. Narang, SK. Child abuse: Social and medicolegal issues. https://www.uptodate.com/contents/child-abuse-social-and-medicolegal-issues?topicRef=6607&source=see_link#H6. 2/18/18.

3. Recognize the signs. Polaris Project. 2018. https://polarisproject.org/human-trafficking/recognize-signs. Accessed on 5/25/2018.

CONFLICT OF INTEREST[1,2]

A conflict of interest can arise if there are financial relationships with the pharmaceutical industry, medical device companies, laboratories, and/or imaging centers whereby the relationship can affect the provision of health care to patients. Conflicts of interest can negatively affect patient care and impede evidence-based medical practice.

The AAPA provides a statement about conflict of interest and states that PAs should put patient care above material gain and that PAs are ethically obligated to disclose any potential or actual conflicts of interest to their patients.

Some examples of potential conflicts of interest include:

- Accepting gifts from pharmaceutical or medical device companies

- Speaking or writing on behalf of an industry

- Engaging in a financial relationship with an industry or facility

Always err on the side of disclosure when there is any concern about a possible conflict of interest. Most hospital and healthcare systems will also require you to sign a conflict of interest statement upon hire and annually, particularly if the facility is affiliated with an academic medical center.

References:

1. Institute of Medicine (US) Committee on Conflict of Interest in Medical Research, Education, and Practice; Lo B, Field MJ, editors. Conflict of Interest in Medical Research, Education, and Practice. Washington (DC): National Academies Press (US); 2009. 6, Conflicts of Interest and Medical Practice. Available from: https://www.ncbi.nlm.nih.gov/books/NBK22944/

2. AAPA. (2013). Guidelines for Ethical Conduct for the Physician Assistant Profession. https://www.aapa.org/wp-content/uploads/2017/02/16-EthicalConduct.pdf

IMPAIRED PROVIDER[1,2,3,4]

Impairment is defined as the inability to practice medicine with reasonable safety and skill. Impairment can occur due to a physical condition, a mental health condition, and addiction. However, having a physical disease or illness does not necessarily mean the person will be impaired. Disease or illness that causes adverse effects on motor or cognitive skills can cause impairment. The American Medical Association also identifies disruptive behavior as a source of impairment if it interferes with patient care. Disruptive behavior may be due to an underlying disorder, so a diagnostic evaluation is recommended.

The AAPA clearly states that PAs have an ethical responsibility to identify and assist impaired members of the health care team. Most state medical societies and medical boards will have either voluntary or mandatory tracks for impaired PAs and physicians. Criteria for referral could include knowledge or suspicion of illicit drug or excessive alcohol use, behaviors that are concerning for patient and public safety, and known or suspected psychiatric illness that is insufficiently treated.

Voluntary tracks are available to PAs and physicians who self-identify as needing assistance. Safeguards are in place to ensure compliance with treatment, and if non-compliance occurs, a report to the state medical board may be initiated. Mandated tracks are required by state medical boards, and non-compliance could result in revocation or suspension of a medical license.

Remember that burn-out can occur at any time during the course of a career. Surveys and reports from around the country indicate that healthcare provider burnout is double that of other industries. Identifying the early signs and intervening early is critical. The symptoms of burnout include depersonalization, a diminished sense of accomplishment, cynicism, loss of fulfillment, and emotional exhaustion. Healthcare providers who experience burnout have higher rates of depression, suicide, and substance abuse, and are at greater risk of committing a medical error.

Burnout occurs largely because of factors outside of a healthcare provider's control. Electronic medical records, long work hours, and conflicts between work and home and within the workplace are often cited as reasons for burnout. Identifying the symptoms of burnout individually or in others on the healthcare team necessitates referral to a professional trained in the identification and management of burnout.

References:

1. AAPA. (2013). Guidelines for Ethical Conduct for the Physician Assistant Profession. https://www.aapa.org/wp-content/uploads/2017/02/16-EthicalConduct.pdf

2. Dzau, VJ, Kirck, DG, and Nasca, TJ. To care is human: Collectively confronting the clinician-burnout crisis. *N Engl J Med* 2018; 378:312-314. DOI: 10.1056/NEJMp1715127

3. Federation of State Medical Boards. (2011). Policy on Physician Impairment. http://www.fsmb.org/globalassets/advocacy/policies/physician-impairment.pdf

4. Wright, AA and Katz, IT. Beyond burnout: Redesigning care to restore meaning and sanity for physicians. *N Engl J Med* 2018; 378:309-311. DOI: 10.1056/NEJMp1716845

INFORMED CONSENT AND REFUSAL PROCESS [1,2]

Informed consent is based on the moral and legal premise of patient autonomy. This means that the patient has the right to make decisions about his/her own health and medical conditions. For many types of interactions (for example, a physical exam), **implied consent** is assumed, but the PA should still seek verbal permission to perform a physical examination on a patient. For more invasive tests or treatments with significant risks or alternatives, obtain **explicit (written) consent**. Many health systems will have their own consents. If a patient refuses medical treatment, document in the progress note that the patient refused treatment, and have the patient sign an "Against Medical Advice" form as well.

There are four components of informed consent:

• The patient must have the **capacity** (or ability) to make the decision.

• The medical provider must disclose information on the treatment, test, or procedure, including the expected **risks, benefits, and alternatives**, and the probability that the benefits and risks will occur.

• The patient must comprehend the relevant information.

• The must voluntarily grant consent, **without coercion or duress**

The following components should be discussed and included in the written consent form:

• An **explanation of the medical condition** that warrants the test, procedure, or treatment.

• An **explanation of the purpose and benefits** of the proposed test, procedure, or treatment.

• An **explanation or description** of the proposed test, procedure, or treatment, including possible complications or adverse events.

• A **description of alternative treatments**, procedures, or tests, if any, and their relative benefits and risks.

• A discussion of the **consequences** of not accepting the test, procedure, or treatment.

If, because of intoxication, injury, illness, or severe emotional stress, it may be decided that a patient does not have decision-making capacity. The patient may not be able to refuse treatment in those cases. The law presumes that the average reasonable person would consent to treatment in most emergencies to prevent permanent disability or death. Decision-making capacity is often referred to by the legal term competency. It is one of the most important components of informed consent.

The components of decision-making capacity are as follows:

• The ability to **understand the options**.

• The ability to **understand the consequences** of choosing each of the options.

• The ability to **evaluate the personal cost and benefit** of each of the consequences and relate them to your own set of values and priorities.

Most states give decision-making authority to un-emancipated minors with decision-making capacity (mature minors) who are seeking treatment for certain medical conditions, including drug/alcohol abuse/addiction, pregnancy, sexually transmitted infections, and contraception. There are more limitations for elective abortions, so know the state's statutes.

Sometimes, there can be confusion between the terms capacity and competence. It is important to know the difference as one can be determined by a PA, but the other must be determined by the courts.

Capacity: decision-making ability, determined by any attending physician/PA:

• Assess capacity even when patient agrees with your recommendations.

• Consult psychiatry, ethics committee, and/or risk management in difficult situations.

• Questions you can ask to determine capacity:

   o "What do you think is wrong with you?"

   o "What do you think the treatment will do for you?"

   o "What do you think will happen if you do not do what is suggested?"

   o "How would your life be affected if you experienced side effects or benefits of treatment?"

   o "How did you come to reach your decision about your options?"

Competence: capacity to make medical decision, determined by the courts.

Sometimes it is necessary to call for a psychiatric consultation when you encounter difficult situations. In certain circumstances, it may be necessary to place a 72-hour legal hold on a patient deemed to be a danger to themselves or others. Often, patients who require a 72-hour hold have an underlying psychiatric disorder, including substance abuse.

The MacArthur Competence Assessment Tools for Treatment (MacCAT-T) is regarded as the **gold standard** for capacity assessment and can be found here: http://ps.psychiatryonline.org/doi/pdf/10.1176/ps.48.11.1415

References:

1. Jonsen AR, Siegler M, Winslade WJ. Clinical Ethics: *A Practical Approach to Ethical Decisions in Clinical Medicine*, 8th Ed. 2015; New York: McGraw-Hill Education.

2. Mappes TA, DeGrazia D. *Biomedical Ethics*, 7th Ed. 2010; New York: McGraw-Hill Education.

LIVING WILL, ADVANCE DIRECTIVES, ORGAN DONATION, CODE STATUS, DO NOT RESUSCITATE, DO NOT INTUBATE, MEDICAL POWER OF ATTORNEY

In 1990, a federal law called the ***Patient Self-Determination Act*** was passed.[1] This requires hospitals and other health care facilities to provide patients with a written summary that includes rights to make health care decisions and the hospital's policies regarding advanced directives. It also requires that upon admission to a health care facility, the patient be asked if they have an advance directive; it is up to the patient to provide the document to the facility. In addition, the health care facility cannot discriminate against any patient based on an advance directive. Some states will require patients to use a specific form, while others will allow a patient to write their own.

Advanced directives fall into two broad categories: **instructive and proxy**.

Instructive directives:

• Allows for patient preferences regarding particular treatments.

    o ***Living wills*** are the most common examples of instructive directives, and would supersede instructions given by a proxy (i.e. durable power of attorney for health care).

• A living will provides specific instructions to health care providers and the patient's families and friends about the patient's wishes regarding end-of-life care, including CPR, intubation, organ donation, enteral or parenteral feeding, and palliative care.

• Do Not Attempt Resuscitation (DNAR), Do Not Resuscitate (DNR), Do Not Intubate (DNI) orders can be signed by a PA.

    o Other types of instructive directives are "no transfusion" and mental health directives.

Proxy directives:

• Allows for the designation of a spokesperson for the patient.

    o ***The Durable Power of Attorney for Health Care*** (DPAHC) is the most common proxy directive. If a patient has a living will, the living will supersede the DPAHC.

The American Heart Association recommends that patients who experience cardiac arrest should receive resuscitative measures unless there is a valid DNR order, or if resuscitative efforts would be futile in the case of irreversible death (i.e. decapitation). Other reasons to withhold CPR include anencephaly and extreme prematurity (<23 weeks gestation).

References:

1. The Patient Self-Determination Act (PSDA). acs.org. https://www.cancer.org/treatment/finding-and-paying-for-treatment/understanding-financial-and-legal-matters/advance-directives/patient-self-determination-act.html

2. The American Heart Association. Part 3: Ethical Issues. https://eccguidelines.heart.org/index.php/circulation/cpr-ecc-guidelines-2/part-3-ethical-issues/

CARING FOR PATIENTS WITH COGNITIVE IMPAIRMENT

Cognitive impairment is often seen in patients with dementia and delirium, but can also occur in patients with developmental disabilities, patients who have had a stroke, or patients with a traumatic brain injury. It is important to recognize cognitive impairment in a patient to avoid causing any harm and to ensure proper medical surrogacy. Medicare recognizes the importance of a thorough assessment of cognitive function as well as the development of a care plan to fit the patient's and caregivers' needs.[1] As such, starting in January 2018, the CPT code is 99483 and replaces the previous HCPCS code G0505.[2] **The CPT code 99483 allows PAs to bill for cognitive impairment assessment and care planning.** Use of the 99483/G0505 code requires nine elements be assessed and documented.

History and physical examination, including a cognitive evaluation using the Mini-CogTM or the Short MoCA. The Mini-Cog can be found here: https://www.alz.org/documents_custom/minicog.pdf and the Short MoCA can be found here: http://www.mocatest.org/.

• Functional assessment of the ability to perform activities of daily living, as well as ability to make decisions.

• Staging of cognitive impairment or dementia.

• Medication review and reconciliation.

• Evaluation of behavioral and/or neuropsychiatric issues.

• Safety assessment.

• Caregiver assessment, including identifying caregivers.

• Advanced planning, including end-of-life and palliative care needs and wants.

• A documentation of the provider's medical decision-making, ranked as moderate or complex.

The creation of a care plan can be billed separately, at a different visit if needed, but the care plan must include any referrals, including community resource referrals, and how neuropsychiatric/behavioral issues will be addressed. In addition, the care plan must be shared with the patient/caregiver.

The Alzheimer's Association created a Cognitive Assessment Toolkit that can be found here: https://www.alz.org/documents_custom/141209-CognitiveAssessmentToo-kit-final.pdf

References:

1. Alzheimer's Association. 2017. Cognitive impairment care planning. https://www.alz.org/careplanning/

2. Don't miss these four important coding changes for 2018. American Academy of Family Physicians. In Practice Blog. https://www.aafp.org/journals/fpm/blogs/inpractice/entry/four_important_coding_changes_for_2018.html. Accessed 5/1/2018.

PATIENT/PROVIDER RIGHTS AND RESPONSIBILITIES

The right to have access to and maintain privacy of medical records is guaranteed under federal law. Other patient protections involve health care insurance, including the right to preventive health care, to not be charged higher fees for a preexisting condition, and to not be unenrolled from an insurance plan if the patient becomes ill. The American Hospital Association[1] first developed a Patient Bill of Rights in 1973 and was later revised in 1992. In 2010, the Bill of Rights was expanded to include protections regarding health insurance coverage in light of the Affordable Care Act.[2] The law allows patients the following rights:

• To receive respectful, considerate, and linguistically appropriate care.

• To obtain understandable and current information about their diagnosis, treatment, and prognosis.

• To be informed about their medical condition, the risks and benefits of treatment, and appropriate alternatives, except in the case of a medical emergency.

• To be informed about the financial impact of their medical decisions, if known.

• To know the identity of every person involved in their care, including PAs and students.

• To consent or refuse treatment at any stage of care without fear of retribution, but must be provided with information regarding the potential medical consequences of consent or refusal.

• To have an advance directive, including a living will, health care proxy, durable power of attorney for health care, or surrogate; and that the health care provider or hospital will honor the directive.

• To have privacy, with access to their records limited to those involved in their care or clearly designated by the patient, and with assurances that information will be kept private.

• To have confidentiality of their records, unless abuse is suspected, in which case all members of the health care team are mandated reporters.

• To access their medical records.

• To obtain reasonable care and services as indicated by medical urgency.

• To not be transferred to another facility unless the patient requests the transfer or when care cannot be provided at the current facility, but only when the patient is stable, and only if the transfer is accepted by the second institution. (See EMTALA under Medico-legal Issues below).

• To ask about any potential conflict of interest between the health care providers, the institutions, and payers that could influence the treatment of the patient.

• To consent or decline participation in clinical research without fear of retribution, with an appropriate informed consent process.

• To have continuity of care, as medically appropriate.

• To receive notice of office and hospital policies related to patient care, including patient and provider responsibilities.

• To be informed of processes to resolve disputes and conflicts.

• To be made aware of the potential charges and payment methods.

• To receive full disclosure of their insurance plan in plain language.

Patient responsibilities[1]

Patients also have responsibilities to their health care providers. This includes providing accurate information about their medical, surgical, and social history, including any medications, illicit drugs, alcohol, or tobacco use. Patients are responsible for understanding that lifestyle choices may positively or negatively impact their health and treatment of illness. Patients must also ask for clarification or more information if they do not understand any element of their visit or care plan. Patients must disclose any barriers to following directions for treatment, including ability to fill prescriptions, and patients must provide accurate insurance information, if covered under any insurance plan. Finally, patients must be considerate of other patients, health care providers, and other staff in the office or hospital.

Providers' rights and responsibilities[3]

Health care providers also have specific rights and responsibilities to their patients. The AAPA maintains that all PAs should act both morally and legally. While the law represents a minimum standard of acceptable behavior, ethical principles demand the highest standard of behavior. The AAPA created a bulleted statement of values for the profession.[3]

These are:

• PAs hold as their primary responsibility the health, safety, welfare, and dignity of all human beings.

• PAs uphold the tenets of patient autonomy, beneficence, nonmaleficence, and justice.

• PAs recognize and promote the value of diversity.

• PAs treat equally all persons who seek their care.

• PAs hold in confidence the information shared in the course of practicing medicine.

• PAs assess their personal capabilities and limitations, striving always to improve their medical practice.

• PAs actively seek to expand their knowledge and skills, keeping abreast of advances in medicine.

• PAs work with other members of the health care team to provide compassionate and effective care of patients.

• PAs use their knowledge and experience to contribute to an improved community.

• PAs respect their professional relationship with physicians.

• PAs share and expand knowledge within the profession.

In addition, the AAPA also states that "the patient–PA relationship is also a patient–PA–physician relationship," reinforcing the concept of the importance of functioning as a team. Furthermore, PAs must also provide appropriate and unbiased information so that patients can make informed decisions; disclose to their collaborating physician any medical errors that may have occurred during the course of treating a patient; and must be aware of any conflicts of interest and properly disclose those conflicts to involved parties.

The American Academy of Physician Assistants publishes Guidelines for Ethical Conduct for the Physician Assistant Profession and can be found here: https://www.aapa.org/wp-content/uploads/2017/02/16-EthicalConduct.pdf.

References:

1. The American Hospital Association. (2018). The patient care partnership: Understanding expectations, rights and responsibilities. https://www.aha.org/system/files/2018-01/aha-patient-care-partnership.pdf

2. Centers for Medicare and Medicaid Services https://www.cms.gov/CCIIO/Programs-and-Initiatives/Health-Insurance-Market-Reforms/Patients-Bill-of-Rights.html

3. Guidelines for the Ethical Conduct for the Physician Assistant Profession. aapa.org. https://www.aapa.org/wp-content/uploads/2017/02/16-EthicalConduct.pdf. Accessed 5/15/2018.

Further information:

American Academy of Physician Assistants. https://www.aapa.org/wp-content/uploads/2017/02/16-

EthicalConduct.pdf

PROVIDING PATIENT ADVICE AND EDUCATION RELATED TO END-OF-LIFE DECISIONS

While medical ethics strongly supports patient autonomy, sometimes physicians and PAs need to balance autonomy (the right to decide for one's self) with **paternalism** (the healthcare provider decides for the patient even when the patient has the capacity to decide for him/herself), specifically as it relates to end-of-life decisions. The term **"palliative paternalism"** has been used to describe how the health care provider can guide end-of-life discussions.[1] It is the provider's responsibility to review the patient's understanding of the disease process; how the progression of disease effects the patient's quality of life and how the patient defines quality of life; benefits and risks of medical interventions, including possible pain or adverse outcomes with each intervention; and provide a reasonable prognosis with and without treatments, including survival and potential disability.

Telling the truth to a patient who is dealing with a terminal illness is imperative. The way in which this information is disclosed should be well thought-out and appropriate to each patient's circumstances. **Medical futility** is a term used to describe excessive medical intervention that would not change the outcome of the disease process. In patients facing a terminal disease, it is important to remember that discussions around pain control should not center around the futility of the patient's disease process, but rather the reassurance that the patient's pain will be controlled.

As such, assessing the need for pain control is central to discussions regarding end-of-life care. Each patient should be allowed to openly express their need for and expectations regarding pain medication and other symptoms common at the end of life, such as difficulty breathing. Opioids and adjuvant medications commonly used in hospice and end-of-life care should never be rationed.

In end-of-life care planning, pain control must be a priority and the patient assured that his or her pain will be controlled, even if it may hasten death. However, the patient and caregiver must be made aware that pain control measures will not be used solely to hasten death.[2]

Patients at the end of life will voluntarily cease to eat and drink. This is a normal process in a dying patient. Often, a patient will have a Do Not Resuscitate (DNR) order, but sometimes an order to Allow Natural Death will be in place.[3]

The term hospice care can be used interchangeably with palliative care. **Hospice**

and palliative care incorporate the patient's spiritual, religious, and emotional issues in care planning. In this sense, it is a team-based service. Palliative care simply means offering the patient relief of symptoms with no expectation that the disease will be cured. To qualify for hospice care, a patient should have a prognosis of six months or less, but more often patients with chronic, long-term diseases such as dementia are being referred earlier as it is difficult to say when a patient with a disease such as dementia may die. Reauthorization of hospice services can be accomplished with a simple nurse visit and adequate documentation.

An end of life checklist should include the following:

- Have wishes for end-of-life care been discussed?

- Is there a power of attorney for financial and health care decisions?

- Is palliative or hospice appropriate?

- Is there a DNR?

- Is there a Physician Order for Life-sustaining Treatment?

Communicating with patients and their loved ones about end-of-life decisions can be difficult, but providing open communication is necessary to facilitate patients' understanding of their prognosis and options, and the earlier the discussion is had, the better the outcome for patients and families.

As a PA, you will likely encounter patients who are actively dying. The process of dying is not a defining event, but rather a series of smaller events or milestones leading up to the patient's final breath. It is important to prepare family members and other caregivers for this process and reassure them that what is happening is normal. **The physiologic changes** seen in terminally ill patients that tend to be harbingers of death include the following[3]:

- The skin changes color and sometimes becomes mottled.

- The patient will spend more time sleeping, may become unarousable, or obtunded.

- Bowel and bladder incontinence commonly occurs, and urine output will decrease.

- Pulmonary congestion increases as oral mucosal secretions thicken and the patient becomes less able to cough.

- Psychomotor agitation or restlessness is common.

• The breathing pattern will change, alternating between periods of "normal" breathing with rapid, shallow breathing and slower breathing, sometimes having apneic periods of up to one minute.

During the active dying process, it is not uncommon for patients to begin emotionally detaching from friends and family.

Many patients will claim that they see a person who has already died, that they know when they are going to die, and that they feel an angel in the room[3]. It is important to continue to offer support to the patient and their friends and family during this period and offer reassurance that what is happening is normal. Finally, every person grieves in their own way. Be respectful of the patient, friends, and family members as they navigate through the process. Hospice and palliative care offers spiritual and religious assistance, so do not be afraid to call on members of the team to assist someone who may seem to be struggling and could potentially use some help.

References:

1.   Roeland E, Cain J, Onderdonk C, Kerr K, Mitchell W, Thornberry K. When open-ended questions don't work: the role of palliative paternalism in difficult medical decisions. *J Palliat Med.* 2014 Apr;17(4):415-20. Epub 2014 Mar 3

2.   LeBlanc, TW and James Tulsky, J. Discussing goals of care. https://www.uptodate.com/contents/discussing-goals-of care?search=end%20 of%20life%20discussion&source=search_result&selectedTitle=1~150&usage_type=defa ult&display_rank=1

3.   Lee BC. Chapter 51: End-of-life issues. In Ballweg R, et al. *Physician assistant: A guide to clinical practice.* 5th ed. Philadelphia, PA: Elsevier; 2013.

Further reading:

AARP. Prepare to Care. https://assets.aarp.org/www.aarp.org_/articles/foundation/aa66r2_care.pdf

COMMON MEDICOLEGAL ISSUES

EMTALA

The Emergency Medical Treatment and Active Labor Act, also known as EMTALA, was enacted by the U.S. Congress in 1986 as a response to many hospitals "dumping" Medicaid and uninsured patients on public hospitals.[1] This piece of federal legislation applies to patients who are treated at any health care facility that receives payments from the U.S. Department of Health and Human Services (HHS). EMTALA requires all patients receive an adequate medical screening examination (MSE) that evaluates the presence of a medical emergency. PAs can, by law, perform the MSE, but the facility must specifically have PAs identified as credentialed providers to perform the MSE.[2] The medical screening examination must not be delayed to inquire about insurance coverage or ability to pay.

• **A medical condition that is defined as emergent is** "a condition manifesting itself by acute symptoms of sufficient severity (including severe pain) such that the absence of immediate medical attention could reasonably be expected to result in placing the individual's health [or the health of an unborn child] in serious jeopardy, serious impairment to bodily functions, or serious dysfunction of bodily organs."[1]

If a patient is found to have a medical emergency, he/she must receive treatment, including stabilizing treatment, regardless of their ability to pay. If a patient presents in active labor, she must be delivered at that facility unless a clear indication for a transfer to another facility exists.

Hospitals that have specialized services and capabilities are obligated under EMTALA to accept patient transfers from hospitals if the transferring hospital lacks the ability to adequately treat the patient's emergency condition.[1] If a hospital receives a patient from another facility that may be in violation of EMTALA, the hospital is required to report the possible violation to the CMS.

PAs must be mindful of the legal requirements regarding the transfer of patients from facility to facility. If a patient requests a transfer, the transfer must be in written form and signed by the patient. The transferring provider must receive acceptance of the transfer and appropriately document in the patient's chart that acceptance of the transfer was obtained. In addition, the transferring facility is responsible to transport the patient to the other facility. If a patient is medically unstable, the provider must document the reasons for the transport, including the risks and benefits of the transfer.[1] Maternal-fetal conditions that may necessitate a transfer to a facility with specialized services include:

- Preterm labor and preterm premature rupture of membranes

- Severe preeclampsia or eclampsia

- Bleeding disorders

- Fetal anomalies

- Multiple gestation

Pregnant patients with co-morbid medical conditions may also require a transfer to a facility with specialized services.[1]

Some of these conditions include:

- Trauma

- Acute surgical condition

- Sepsis

- Cardiovascular or respiratory diseases

- Coagulopathies

- Neurological diseases

- Psychiatric diseases, including illicit drug addiction and overdose

Transfer to another facility may not be advisable in certain circumstances. For example, if there is no appropriate transfer vehicle for the patient, if weather or road conditions are hazardous, if delivery of the fetus is anticipated prior to arrival at the receiving hospital, severe fetal anomalies that result in death of the neonate, and any condition where a possible delay in delivery of the fetus would result in unnecessary death or significant damage to the mother or fetus.[1]

According to CMS, PAs can determine if a patient is in active or false labor if they are providing the examination within their scope of practice as outlined by the hospital.[2] PAs can take emergency room call and determine medical necessity. PAs can also order the transfer of a patient to another facility, but the PA must consult with a physician first, and the physician must co-sign the order.[2]

Violations of EMTALA can result in significant monetary fines and revocation of provider agreements. It may also result in secondary civil suits. In a review of litigation between 2002 and 2015[3], 192 settlements occurred. The monetary fines totaled $6,357,000. Over 95% of settlements were against hospitals. The most common reasons for EMTALA violations were failure to properly screen and failure to stabilize the patient. Approximately 20% of violations were due to inappropriate transfers, including failure to transfer to a facility with more specialized services.

EMTALA applies to urgent care facilities that are owned by a hospital or are part of a joint venture with a hospital or hospital system. EMTALA also applies to free-standing emergency departments.

References:

1.   American College of Emergency Physicians. (2016). EMTALA. https://www.acep.org/news-media-top banner/emtala/#sm.0001hfrce 91391e1msn4o76h6ce4i

2.   American Academy of Physician Assistants. (2017). EMTALA and physician assistants. https://www.aapa.org/wp content/uploads/2017/01 /EMTALA_and_Physician_Assistants.pdf

3.   Zuabi N, Weiss LD, Langdorf MI. Emergency Medical Treatment and Labor Act (EMTALA) 2002-15: Review of Office of Inspector General Patient Dumping Settlements. West *J Emerg Med.* 2016 May; 17(3):245-251. Published online 2016 May. doi: 10.5811/westjem.2016.3.29705

Health Insurance Portability and Accountability Act (HIPAA)[1]

The HHS issued the Standards for Privacy of Individually Identifiable Health Information, also known as the "Privacy Rule," to elucidate requirements of the Health Insurance Portability and Accountability Act (HIPAA) in 1996. The Office of Civil Rights, within the HHS, is charged with enforcing the Rule. The Privacy Rule addresses the use and disclosure of personal health information by covered entities. It also outlines an individual's right to privacy and how personal health information is used. The Privacy Rule was modified in 2002, and in 2003, HHS published the Security Rule. The Security Rule was established to protect the integrity, availability, and confidentiality of electronic protected health information.

The Privacy Rule was intended to protect a person's health information while still allowing some sharing of information that would benefit the individual's and the public's health. Here are some important terms to know regarding HIPAA and the Privacy Rule.

- **Protected health information (PHI):**

    o Individually identifiable health information, be it electronic, on paper, or oral.

    o Includes information such as patient demographics, past/present/future medical or mental health condition(s), and financial information, including insurance data.

    o Patient demographics includes personal identifiers, such as date of birth, name, address, and even Social Security number.

- **Covered entity and business associates:**

    o All covered entities and business associates must comply with HIPAA standards.

    o Covered entities include individual health care providers, health plans, and health care clearinghouses.

    o Business associates include individuals or organizations with whom a covered entity contracts, such as medical billing, utilization review, administrative functions, and legal services.

- **National Provider Identifier (NPI):**

  o The NPI is a HIPAA standard.

  o Covered health entities, including PAs, must register and use their NPI for administrative and financial transactions.

  o The NPI is a 10-digit number that does not allow for an identifier, such as medical specialty or state in which one resides.
  Information on how to register or search the registry can be found here: https://nppes.cms.hhs.gov/#/ and https://npiregistry.cms.hhs.gov/

The Security Rule helps protect electronic PHI. Compliance mandates that covered entities protect against threats to the security of PHI and inappropriate use of PHI. It also requires compliance by the covered entity's employees and must demonstrate evidence of employee training. Covered entities must engage in ongoing risk analyses to potential threats to electronic PHI and maintain security protections. The Security Rule also mandates that all covered entities designate an individual who is charged with overseeing security of electronic PHI, including developing, refining, and enforcing policies and procedures related to electronic PHI. Security of workplaces and electronic devices must be well-defined and enforced, and technical safeguards must be utilized in order to protect all electronic PHI.

Health information can be shared without an individual's authorization under certain circumstances. A hospital or health care provider may use PHI about a patient:

- In consultation with other providers in order to form a treatment plan.

- In order to bill insurance for payment of services.

- When referring to a specialist who requires the patient's PHI prior to evaluation.

- When transferring a patient to a skilled nursing facility or other facility.

- When specimens, such as tissue and blood samples, are sent to an external laboratory.

Covered entities are required to establish policies and procedures regarding its use of PHI. For example, medical providers have limited access to patients' PHI in that they may only access information about patients if they are involved in the care of the patient. Providers who access information about any other patient, including themselves and family members, are in clear violation of the Privacy Rule and may be subject to termination.

Covered entities may choose to develop a consent process regarding its use of PHI, but only if the use of PHI does not require formal authorization under the Privacy Rule. A covered entity must adhere to a patient's request regarding how the patient wants to receive personal health information, such as leaving messages on voice mail or for whom information about the patient can be shared. Covered entities must also notify patients of their privacy practices regarding the use of PHI.

The Genetic Information Nondiscrimination Act (GINA) was enacted in 2008. The purpose of GINA is to protect an individual from discrimination based upon genetic information. Covered entities must not use or disclose genetic information for any other purpose than in directly providing patient care. Thus, a covered entity must not disclose or use genetic information for financial purposes.

Compliance violations can result in criminal and civil penalties. The Office of Civil Rights investigates any potential violation and if the violation may result in criminal charges, the Department of Justice will intervene.

Criminal penalties:

Violation	Penalty
"Knowingly violate"	up to $50,000 and one year in prison
"False pretense"	increase of fines up to $100,000 and up to 5 years in prison
"Intent to use PHI for personal financial gain, commercial advantage, or malice"	up to $250,000 and 10 years in prison

Civil penalties:

HIPAA Violation	Minimum Penalty	Maximum Penalty
"Unknowing"	$100 per violation; max $25,000 annually;	$50,000 per violation; max $1.5 million annually
"Reasonable Cause"	$1,000 per violation; max $100,000 for repeat violations	$50,000 per violation; max $1.5 million annually
"Willful neglect" (corrected within required time period)	$10,000 per violation; $250,000 max annually	$50,000 per violation; max $1.5 million annually
"Willful neglect" (not corrected within required time period)	$50,000 per violation; max $1.5 million annually	$50,000 per violation; max $1.5 million annually

Summary:

Personal health information includes information about patients that are alive and deceased, and includes billing information, patient identifiers on specimens, intravenous bags, medical record data, and even pictures of patients. Before any PHI is used, it is necessary to ask if the information is necessary. If the information is specifically for patient care or billing, it is probably safe in accessing it. Remember that personal health information must never be used on any social media platform. Tagging at a healthcare facility and posting about a patient, even if the patient is not named, can still present problems. Also, never post pictures of patients or anything else in a healthcare facility that has any type of identifier.

Reference:

1.   HIPAA for Professionals. United States Department of Health and Human Services. 2017. hhs.gov. https://www.hhs.gov/hipaa/for-professionals/index.html. Accessed 5/10/2018.

MEDICAL MALPRACTICE

Being named in a medical malpractice suit is perhaps one of the biggest fears as PAs. Common reasons for PAs to be named in a suit include[1]:

- Failure to diagnose appropriately.

- Failure to perform an adequate exam.

- Failure to be adequately supervised.

- Failure to provide a timely referral.

- Failure to document appropriately.

- Failure to communicate appropriately.

Most of these reasons can be minimized or even prevented with careful attention to detail and incorporating basic risk management strategies. Good documentation in the medical record provides the reader with details about what was done, what was ordered, and what was prescribed. Excellent documentation allows the reader insight into the thought process as one moves through the history, the physical examination, ancillary testing, diagnoses, and plans. It is a good idea to document medical decision-making in a narrative, particularly when dealing with complicated patients.

Other important actions include[1]:

- Document all conversations with a patient, including phone calls.

- Always date and sign entries in the medical record.

- Never delete anything from the medical record. If something is done in error in an electronic health record, create an addendum.

- If your practice uses paper charts, never use anything to "white-out" any element of the chart. If you make an error in the record, put a single line through the error, initial it, date it, and write "error" next to the error.

- Avoid using abbreviations.

- Do not take shortcuts. The few minutes saved by cutting corners could cost you dearly.

• Be as specific as possible when documenting the history and physical examination findings. Use the patient's words in quotations when necessary.

• Do not cut and paste text from one entry into another.

While the SOAP note format must still be followed, a new addition adds an ER to SOAP, making the mnemonic SOAPER[1]. The E stands for Educate and the R stands for Response.

E: Educate. Examples: The patient was educated about the importance of taking his medications every day as instructed; the patient was educated on the importance of following up with her primary care provider within 24 – 48 hours and to return to the emergency room if symptoms worsen or persist.

R: Response. Example: The patient was given both verbal and written instructions on the diagnosis, the treatment plan, and when and with whom to follow up, and the patient verbalized understanding of instructions.

Once an error has been realized, several steps must occur.[1]

• Disclosure the error. Follow state laws regarding apologies. Apologizing does not admit guilt or wrong-doing. Convey empathy and let them know there will be an investigation about how the error occurred. Do not shift blame on to anyone else, try to offer a defense, or make excuses.

• Notify the risk manager and collaborating physician.

• Do not discuss the case with anyone else, particularly outside the healthcare facility.

PAs are required to have medical malpractice insurance. Most PAs are covered by their employers, but there are options to obtain supplemental individual coverage as well. For example, the AAPA offers supplemental medical malpractice insurance.

There are two types of malpractice insurance, occurrence and claims-made. Occurrence insurance will cover you during the time you had the coverage independent of when the claim is filed. For example, if the PA leaves an employer and take a new position and is covered under a different malpractice insurance carrier, and the PA is subsequently named in a suit whereby the alleged offense occurred during the time at the previous employer, occurrence insurance will cover the PA. Claims-made coverage, however, will not cover the PA unless tail coverage exists.

Malpractice insurance policies will offer limits of coverage. Typical amounts are $100,000 - $300,000 for each claim made against the PA during the time of coverage under the policy, and $1 million - $3 million for all claims made against the PA during the time of coverage under the policy. If the PA is involved in surgery, trauma, emergency medicine, cardiac catheterization, and/or obstetrics, insurance premiums are likely to be higher.

In order for a claim to be considered under **malpractice laws**, it must demonstrate the following:

- the PA's interaction with the patient falls outside the accepted **standard of care**;

- the patient was harmed as a result of the action;

- quantifiable damages occurred.

Medical negligence claims can be made if the following occurs and it results in harm to the patient and the harm (damages) can be quantified:

- Failure to diagnose.

- Perform unnecessary surgery or invasive procedures.

- Commit surgical errors.

- Failure to follow-up on abnormal labs or imaging.

- Failure to take an adequate history.

- Prescribing the wrong medication, including incorrect dosing that causes harm.

- Discharging a patient from the hospital prematurely and/or fail to follow-up with a patient.

The standard of care is a term used to describe accepted practices and processed used by health care providers in order to treat patients with a disease or illness. Sometimes the standard of care is geographically determined. For example, if a PA is practicing in a rural area without access to telemedicine or stat labs, the action of the PA would be compared with other health care providers working in a similar environment. Standards of care can change over the course of the lifespan. An elderly patient with a shortened life expectancy might not be expected to receive the same care that a young person with a long life expectancy may receive. This is not to say that standards of care defend rationing of health care, but that many factors are considered.

The time limit for filing claims varies by state. If a patient is discovered to have a foreign object left inside after a surgical procedure, the patient has one year after the discovery of the foreign object or ten years from the initial surgery date if the foreign object was not discovered. Each state has their own statute of limitations on claims that can be filed for injuries incurred to the mother or newborn during labor and delivery.

The first step in the process of being named in a malpractice suit is receipt of a notice letter outlying the intent to file suit. Being named as a defendant in a malpractice claim can be stressful, but it is imperative to make sure proper protocols are followed. Immediately notify the collaborating physician(s) and the malpractice insurance carrier. Failure to promptly notify the carrier could result in compromise of coverage.

Never make any alterations to the patient's chart. Remember that in an electronic medical record, everything that is done is time and date stamped, so even the appearance of changing something in the medical record could be used as evidence against the PA. Do not discuss the claim with anyone other than the collaborating physician(s) and the representing attorney. Do not research or discuss the case with people who may be experts.

The next step is the discovery phase. During this phase, attorneys will seek to collect information from all parties involved in the case. Some of the terms used are:

• *Plaintiff*: the person making the claim.

• *Defendant*: the person being sued.

• *Interrogatories*: written questions that must be answered by the defendant.

• *Requests for disclosure*: information about potential witnesses, both lay and expert, and all providers who were involved in the care of the patient.

• *Requests for production*: requests for all documentation that has been written.

• *Requests for admissions*: requests that require an admission or denial.

• *Expert reports*: expert opinions. These must be available to both parties.

• *Depositions*: sessions with attorneys and all who are named in the suit; while done out of the courtroom, sworn testimony is still required. The deposition will be recorded electronically or by a qualified stenographer.

The court will usually recommend *mediation* in order to settle the case out of court. Mediation requires the presence of a qualified person, called a mediator, who is not directly involved in the lawsuit to try and reach settlement without bringing the case to a courtroom. The mediator cannot impose fines or agree with one party over another. All involved parties attend the mediation session, including a representative from the medical malpractice insurance carrier. If the defendant and the plaintiff can agree on a settlement, an agreed motion for nonsuit will be filed in court, and the judge will then respond with an order of nonsuit, meaning that the case has been adequately settled out of court.

Settling does not mean an admission of guilt; in fact, the settlement document can state that the defendants do not admit negligence and that settling out of court simply avoids the time and distress of defending if the suit goes to trial. If mediation does not result in a settlement, the attorney can file a *motion to dismiss* if the plaintiff fails to produce an expert witness report. Sometimes, the plaintiff decides to drop the charges. This is called a voluntary nonsuit. Another outcome from mediation is that the attorney can file a motion for *summary judgment*. This occurs when the attorney challenges the plaintiff to find an expert witness who can validate the claim of negligence. Finally, if no settlement or other motions can be reached, the case will go to court.

Damages can be *compensatory or punitive*. Compensatory damages include medical costs, lost wages, and pain and suffering. Punitive damages generally occur when willful intent has been established. Punitive damages are intended to punish the health care provider.

There are ways to help prevent malpractice suits and all PAs should follow these basic guidelines:

• Document the thought process, including medical decision-making.

• Document that shared decision-making occurred with the patient/the patient's family/the patient's healthcare proxy.

• Document patient and provider expectations and goals.

• Document if the patient disagrees with or refuses treatment or referrals.

• Document during the visit with the patient, when possible.

• Avoid using medical abbreviations. Using abbreviations can cause errors and misunderstandings.

• Communicate with and show concern to the patient/the patient's family/the patient's healthcare proxy. Patients who perceive their healthcare provider to be caring and a good communicator are less likely to file a malpractice suit.

Reference:

1. Cary RM, Cary J. Chapter 36: Medical malpractice and risk management. In Ballweg R, et al. *Physician Assistant: Guide to Clinical Practice*. 5th ed. Philadelphia, PA: Elsevier; 2013.

Bibliography:

Achar, S and Wu, W. How to reduce your malpractice risk. *Fam Pract Manag.* 2012 Jul-Aug;19(4):21-26.

Barry, DB. The physician's guide to medical malpractice. *BUMC Proceedings* 2001;14:109–112

Malpractice insurance basics. The American Academy of Physician Assistants. https://www.aapa.org/career-central/practice-resources/malpractice-insurance-basics/. Accessed 5/10/2018.

What is medical malpractice? The American Board of Professional Liability Attorneys. http://www.abpla.org/what-is-Malpractice. Accessed 5/10/2018.

MEDICAL INFORMATICS

Billing/coding to maintain accuracy and completeness for reimbursement and administrative purposes.

Medical coding uses alphanumeric codes for the evaluation, diagnosis, and management of patients. Codes are also used when billing for medical services. There are three types of coding systems: ICD-10-CM, HCPCS Level II, and CPT®.

ICD-10-CM

The International Classification of Diseases (ICD) is copyrighted by the World Health Organization and has undergone several iterations. The most current is the ICD-10, or 10th revision, and was implemented in October 2015.[1] The ICD-11 revision will be published by the end of 2018.[2] The CM after ICD-10 stands for Clinical Modification. Use of ICD-10 is mandated for all covered entities as defined by HIPAA. ICD codes are diagnostic codes. The 10th revision expands upon previous classifications to include more detailed information about injuries.

The codes have from three to seven characters.[1] Three-character codes are general diagnoses, or category headings, and should be avoided unless further subdivision is impossible. Subdivisions allow for the reporting of specific information about a disease process, including site of disease, laterality, sequelae, signs and symptoms, acute and chronic conditions, syndromes, and even infectious diseases with or without resistance to antibiotics.[1]

The first letter of the code would fall under a specific category. For example, infectious disease category codes fall under A00 – B99, and respiratory disease category codes are J00 – J99.

Another example is for the diagnosis of transient elevations in blood pressure, R03.0. This code is for elevated blood pressure reading without a diagnosis of hypertension, unless the patient has an established diagnosis of hypertension. An anterior wall ST elevation myocardial infarction would be I21.09, but would be further subclassified by intervention, such as 280, discharged alive with cardiac catheterization.

The more specific the coding, the better the chances for appropriate reimbursement. ICD codes can also be used for quality improvement efforts within a practice or health system.

Reference, and for more information:

1. Centers for Disease Control and Prevention. Official guidelines for coding and reporting, FY 2018. https://www.cdc.gov/nchs/data/icd/10cmguidelines_fy2018_final.pdf

2. World Health Organization. Classifications. http://www.who.int /classifications/icd/revision/en/. Accessed on June 19, 2018.

HEALTHCARE COMMON PROCEDURE CODING SYSTEM (HCPCS)

The HCPCS integrates CPT® codes and consists of five-character alpha-numeric codes that covers aspects of medical care not present in CPT® codes. For example, there are HCPCS codes for durable medical equipment, medical supplies, and certain non-physician services, excluding PA services (PA services are billed under CPT® codes and used with ICD-10 codes).

Current Procedural Terminology (CPT®)

Current Procedural Terminology (CPT®) codes were initially established by the American Medical Association (AMA) in 1966. The AMA maintains the copyright on these codes, and updates are completed annually. CPT codes are used for various medical activities, including evaluation and management of patients (E/M), surgery, radiology, laboratory, and anesthesiology. The codes are submitted to insurance companies in order to determine reimbursement for services rendered. The AMA and CMS developed two-character modifiers that help to clarify the procedure.

There are three categories of CPT® codes:

• *Category I:*

Five-digit codes for a service or a procedure. Range is 00100 – 99499.

Evaluation and management codes range from 99201 – 99499.

• *Category II:*

Optional alphanumeric codes for "execution measurement."

• *Category III:*

Provisional codes for developing or new procedures.

Improper billing of services can be considered fraudulent. It is imperative to understand the general principles of documenting the evaluation and management of each patient. Medical record documentation that is clear, concise, and accurate helps to ensure quality of care, appropriate reimbursement for services, and helps other members of the health care team in the care of the patient. Health insurers may require certain documentation for services and may audit charts for appropriateness. Clear, concise, and accurate documentation can also protect against malpractice claims if there is evidence from the note that the evaluation and management of the patient met standards of care and that scope of practice was followed. Always remember that unless it is documented in the record, it never happened. It is also important to document the encounter as soon as possible.

The main reason for denial of medical claims is incomplete or lack of medical record documentation. Sufficient documentation must include a narrative regarding the medical necessity of a hospital admission or surgical procedure, clear documentation regarding care provided and medical decision-making, verify diagnostic results, and concise support for the diagnosis and subsequent decisions made.

Documentation must include the following:

- Reason for encounter.

- Relevant history (includes HPI, PMH, PSH).

- Relevant physical exam findings.

- Prior visits and diagnostics relevant to the encounter.

- Assessment, impression, or diagnosis.

- Plan of care, including referrals.

- Diagnoses and evaluation/management codes must be supported by documentation.

- Name of provider.

- Date of encounter.

Billing for services[1] involves first identifying the visit as new or established. A new patient must not have received medical care from a physician or non-physician provider within the group in the previous three years. An established patient is a patient who has received medical care within the past three years. Evaluation and management services are further categorized by the setting where medical care is provided. Settings include office or outpatient, hospital inpatient, nursing facility, and emergency department.

Categorizing the visit by type of history is a requirement when coding for E/M services.[1] The types of histories are problem focused, expanded problem focused, detailed, and comprehensive. The chief complaint is required in all visits. The others are broken down by the following:

• Problem focused: brief HPI; ROS, past medical, family, and social history when appropriate

• Expanded problem focused: brief HPI, ROS that is problem pertinent, and past medical, family, and social history when appropriate

• Detailed: extended HPI, extended ROS, family and social history that is pertinent

• Comprehensive: extended HPI, complete ROS, and complete past medical, family, and social history

Definitions:

Brief HPI	1 -3 elements
Extended HPI	≥ 4 elements of current HPI or ≥ 3 elements of a chronic condition
Problem-pertinent ROS	System directly related to the problem identified in the HPI
Extended ROS	System directly related to the problem(s) identified in the HPI and a limited number (two to nine) of additional systems.
Complete ROS	System(s) directly related to the problem(s) identified in the HPI plus all additional (minimum of ten) organ systems with pertinent positives and negatives
Pertinent past medical, family, and social history	Review of the history areas directly related to the problem(s) identified in the HPI. The pertinent PFSH must document at least one item from any of the three history areas.
Complete past medical, family, and social history	Review of all three history areas for services that, by their nature, include a comprehensive assessment or reassessment of the patient.

Physical examinations of multiple and single systems are classified as problem-focused, expanded problem focused, detailed, and comprehensive depending upon how many body systems.

• **Multi-system:**

    o Problem focused: examination of 1 -5 elements in ≥ 1 organ system/body area

    o Expanded problem focused: examination of ≥ 6 elements in ≥ 1 organ system/body area

    o Detailed: examination of ≥ 2 elements in ≥ 6 organ systems/body areas; may examine ≥ 12 elements in one or two organ systems/body area

    o Comprehensive: examination of all elements in at least 9 organ systems/body areas

• **Single system:**

    o Problem focused: examination of 1 – 5 elements

    o Expanded problem focused: examination of ≥ 6 elements

    o Detailed: examination of ≥ 12 elements (unless an ophthalmic or psychiatric problem: examination of at least nine elements)

    o Comprehensive: examination of every element

Medical decision-making is documented by complexity in terms of diagnoses and management plans.

Medical decision-making	Number of diagnoses	Complexity of data	Risk of complications, morbidity, and mortality
Straightforward	Minimal	Minimal to none	Minimal
Low complexity	Limited	Limited	Low
Moderate complexity	Multiple	Moderate	Moderate
High complexity	Extensive	Extensive	High

The various levels of medical decision-making correlate with the type of history and physical examination you will perform. The time it should take you to complete the encounter also correlates well with the level of medical decision-making.

Level	CPT code (Established patient)	Time in minutes	History	Physical examination	Medical decision-making
1	99211	5	N/A	N/A	N/A: usually a nurse visit
2	99212	10	Problem-focused	Problem-focused	Straightforward
3	99213	15	Expanded problem-focused	Expanded problem-focused	Low complexity
4	99214	25	Detailed	Detailed	Moderate complexity
5	99215	40	Comprehensive	Comprehensive	Moderate to high complexity

Always remember that unless it is documented, it did not happen. Thus, if one bills for a 99214 visit and there is no documentation that a detailed history and a detailed physical examination were performed, and that moderate complexity medical decision-making was utilized, the code 99214 cannot be used and may constitute fraud.

Reference:

1. Department of Health and Human Services Centers for Medicare & Medicaid Services Evaluation and Management Services. August 2017. https://www.cms.gov/Outreach-and-Education/Medicare-Learning-Network-MLN/MLNProducts/Downloads/eval-mgmt-serv-guide-ICN006764.pdf

THE PHYSICIAN/PA RELATIONSHIP

Professional and clinical limitations, scope of practice, communicating and consulting with the collaborating physician and/or other specialists/consultants.

The PA-physician relationship must be grounded in mutual respect, trust, and open communication. Collaboration demands that PAs provide appropriate communication with physicians and that physicians are available for consultation and assistance when required. Always remember to be cognizant of HIPAA rules and make every effort not to violate a patient's privacy. For example, do not share identifying information about a patient with your collaborating physician in a public area where others may overhear the conversation.

If the PA makes an error in the care of a patient, he or she must disclose the error as soon as possible to the collaborating physician. Disclosing an error to the physician and risk management does not infer negligent or unethical practice but choosing to not disclose an error is considered unethical behavior.[1]

Prompt consultation with other physicians/specialists must be carried out according to HIPAA rules and regulations. Always document in the medical record with whom you are referring the patient and why. Document that the patient is aware of the referral and verbalized understanding of the referral.

Scope of practice[2]

The scope of practice of PAs should be practice and physician specific, not state mandated. Thus, the scope of practice should be decided upon by health care facilities and physicians at the practice level. Prior to employment by a hospital, PAs must apply for clinical privileges, a process called credentialing. It is then up to the medical staff to decide upon the PAs specific scope of practice for that facility. This is the same process that is required of physicians when applying for medical or surgical privileges.

Most states allow PAs to prescribe Schedule II-V medications, but six states currently do not authorize PAs to prescribe Schedule II medications. The level of collaboration and/or supervisory requirements by physicians varies among states. Some states still require physician co-signage of charts, but the percentage of charts varies by state. In addition, some states still limit the number of PAs with whom a physician can either supervise or collaborate.

The **AAPA defines six fundamental aspects of modern PA practice**, including statements regarding supervision, collaboration, and scope of practice of PAs[3].

1. The regulation of PAs by state boards should use the term licensure as opposed to registered or certified. Per the AAPA, licensure implies that the highest levels of professional qualifications have been used.

2. Prescriptive authority should be granted to all nationally certified PAs. This prescriptive authority means that PAs should be able to prescribe Schedule II – V medications, non-scheduled/controlled medications, and medical equipment, such as diabetic shoes. Inability of PAs to have full prescriptive authority interrupts patient care.

3. The scope of practice of PAs should be determined at each practice.

4. The relationship of a PA to the collaborating physician should not be limited by proximity and should not have restrictions or requirements, such as how often the physician must meet with the PA. The AAPA terms this as an adaptable collaboration.

5. Required co-signing of charts should be determined at the practice level and with consideration to the site and the patients being served. Retrospective chart reviews are only one way in which PAs and physicians can communicate, and the AAPA endorses ongoing appropriate communication between PAs and physicians.

6. Restrictions on the number of PAs with whom a physician may collaborate should be practice-level specific. Several physician organizations support this tenet, including the AMA, the Society of Hospital Medicine, and the American College of Emergency Physicians.

There are different ways in which PAs can be supervised by physicians.[5] Prospective supervision occurs when the physician and the PA agree upon the PA's scope of practice. Some states require a written, formal document called a delegation agreement or written agreement that outlines the expectations of the physician and the PA. Concurrent supervision occurs when the supervising physician is present on a daily basis. Within concurrent supervision, there are three subtypes: general, direct, and personal. Finally, there is retrospective supervision whereby the physician performs chart reviews of the PA.

There are different types of physician supervision of PAs. They include:

• **Prospective:** delegation agreement or practice agreement.

- **Retrospective:** chart reviews
- **Concurrent:**

   o General: the physician is available to the PA, either in person or by phone

   o Direct: the physician must be physically present in the facility

   o Personal: the physician must be present while the PA is seeing the patient

The AMA supports the role of the PA as a collaborative provider functioning within the PA's scope of practice but maintains that physicians are ultimately responsible for overseeing the care of patients.[4] Thus, the AMA is opposed to legislation that would authorize PAs to practice medicine independently. However, the AMA supports licensing and the regulation of PAs through state medical boards.

PAs must protect themselves, patients, and collaborating physician(s), by always being cognizant of the delegated scope of practice. If asked to perform an act that is outside one's comfort zone or clearly outside of one's scope of practice, speak up.

References:

1. Guidelines for the Ethical Conduct for the Physician Assistant Profession. aapa.org. https://www.aapa.org/wp-content/uploads/2017/02/16-EthicalConduct.pdf. Accessed 5/15/2018.

2. PAs Scope of Practice. aapa.org. https://www.aapa.org/wp-content/uploads/2017/01/Issue-brief_Scope-of-Practice_0117-1.pdf. Accessed 5/15/2018.

3. Six key elements of a modern PA practice act. aapa.org. https://www.aapa.org/wp-content/uploads/2016/12/Issue_Brief_Six_Key_Elements.pdf. Accessed 5/18/2018.

4. American Medical Association. (2018). Physician assistant scope of practice. https://www.ama-assn.org/sites/default/files/media-browser/public/arc-public/state-law-physician-assistant-scope-practice.pdf. Accessed 5/18/2018.

5. Kohlhepp WC, Brenneman A, VanderMeulen S. Chapter 53: Physician assistants and supervision. In Ballweg R, et al. *Physician Assistant: A Guide to Clinical Practice*. 5th ed. Philadelphia, PA: Elsevier; 2013.

CRITICALLY ANALYZING EVIDENCE-BASED MEDICINE[1,2,3,4]

Carl Heneghen is a Professor of Evidence-based Medicine and Director of the Centre for Evidence Based Medicine at the University of Oxford. He defined evidence-based medicine (EBM) as the "conscientious, explicit, and judicious development and use of current best evidence in making decisions about the care of individual patients."[1]

Evidence-based medicine does not require PAs or other health care providers to engage in bench research or prolonged review of clinical research studies. Rather, EBM helps to inform clinical practice through the application of basic research methods to answer a clinical question. Utilization of the PICO method (see below) is a widely established process to form solid clinical questions. Developing a cogent PICO question is the first step in practicing EBM. The PICO question should be specific so that a quick search of the literature will yield the most relevant results.

A breakdown of the acronym PICO follows:

- **P: patient, problem, or population**

    o summarize the chief complaint, symptom, or disease.

- **I: intervention or indicator**

    o what one wants to do; could be prescribing a medication, ordering a test, or recommending a treatment modality.

- **C: comparison**

    o an alternative to what one wants to do; this can be the gold standard, or it could be nothing.

- **O: outcome or result**

    o what one would like to see happen.

Examples of PICO questions:

Example 1

P: pregnant women with risk factors for preeclampsia

I: taking aspirin during pregnancy

C: not taking aspirin during pregnancy

O: reduction in the incidence of preeclampsia

Clinical question: In pregnant women with risk factors for preeclampsia, does taking aspirin during pregnancy reduce the incidence of preeclampsia?

Example 2

P: patients with fibromyalgia

I: acupuncture

C: not using acupuncture

O: improvement in symptoms

Clinical question: In patients with fibromyalgia, does acupuncture improve symptoms?

Example 3

P: patients with known cardiovascular disease on statin therapy

I: omega-3 fatty acid supplementation

C: not taking omega-3 fatty acid

O: reduction in cardiovascular events

Clinical question: In patients with known cardiovascular disease already on a statin, does the addition of omega-3 fatty acids reduce cardiovascular events?

Once the clinical question has been established, quickly search the literature for the answer. It is best to avoid general search engines such as Google. Get in the habit of using scholarly search engines such as PubMed. Depending upon the clinical question, it may be necessary to focus on specific types of articles or reviews. The evidence is stratified by different levels as described in the chart below. Level 1 Evidence is considered the highest level of evidence, while level 5 is considered the lowest.

Levels of Evidence

Question	Step 1 (Level 1*)	Step 2 (Level 2*)	Step 3 (Level 3*)	Step 4 (Level 4*)	Step 5 (Level 5)
How common is the problem?	Local and current random sample surveys	Systematic review of surveys that allow matching to local circumstances	Local non-random sample	Case-series	N/A
Diagnosis	Systematic reviews	Cross sectional studies	Non-consecutive studies, or studies without consistently applied reference standards	Case-control studies	Mechanistic reasoning*
Prognosis	Systematic reviews	Cohort studies	Cohort study or control arm of randomized trial	Case-series or case control studies, or poor quality prognostic cohort study	N/A
Treatment benefits	Systematic reviews of randomized controlled trials (RCTs)	Randomized trial or observational study	Non-randomized controlled cohort/follow-up study	Case-series, case-control studies, or historically controlled studies	Mechanistic reasoning*
Treatment Harms	Systematic review of randomized trials, case-control studies, n-of-1 trial, or observational study	Randomized trial or observational study	Non randomized controlled cohort/follow-up study if there are sufficient numbers to rule out a common harm; duration of follow-up must be sufficient	Case-series, case-control, or historically controlled studies	Mechanistic reasoning*
Screening	Systematic reviews	Randomized trial	Non -randomized controlled cohort/follow-up study	Case-series, case-control, or historically controlled studies	Mechanistic reasoning*

*Mechanistic reasoning is using the principles of pathophysiology and general knowledge about the scientific method to rule out implausible hypotheses, conclusions, and generalizations.

What is the difference between the different types of studies you can encounter while searching for evidence? What follows is an overview of the types of studies you will find.

- **Meta-analysis:**

  o A systematic review of studies using quantitative methods of analyses.

- **Systematic Review:**

  o A comprehensive summary of studies using critical appraisal and quantitative methods.

- **Randomized Controlled Trial (RCT):**

  o A study where participants are randomized in to a control group or experimental group and followed over a specified period of time.

- **Cohort Study:**

  o Prospective or retrospective study where groups of people who are differentiated in some measurable way (often by exposure to a variable and not exposed to the same variable) are followed over time.

- **Case Controlled Study:**

  o Usually a retrospective study where two groups who are differentiated in a measurable way.

- **Case Series:**

  o A report on a group of patients. No control group is identified.

Thus, systematic reviews and meta-analyses are the highest levels of evidence, while expert opinion is considered the lowest level of evidence. However, when making medical decisions about a patient, it is important to consider the evidence, but also individual patients' values and expectations and your individual expertise about clinical decision-making. There is a difference between disease-oriented and patient-oriented medicine.

- **Disease-oriented medicine:** Outcomes of studies that use surrogate markers of health or disease, such as laboratory values or imaging, that does not necessarily directly impact a patient's quality of life. An example of a disease-oriented outcome is a drug that increases bone mineral density but does not reduce the risk of fractures.

• **Patient-oriented medicine:** Outcomes of studies that are patient-centered, such as symptom improvement, quality of life, mortality, and cost. A patient-oriented outcome that could be practice-changing is called a POEM, or patient-oriented evidence that matters. An example of a patient-oriented outcome is a drug that decreases the risk of myocardial infarction.

Cohort and case control studies are often used to research potential causative factors in disease or health. In 1965, Hill2 developed criteria to help determine causation, and these are still used today. It is important to also use common sense and knowledge of pathophysiology to help rule in or rule out possibilities for causation. This is called **plausibility**. The other criteria are explained below.

• The ***strength of the association*** is a statistical metric expressed as an odds ratio or relative risk. Stronger associations are more likely to be causal.

• ***Consistency of the association*** requires a demonstrable association in different studies and situations. Consistency is associated with causation.

• ***Specificity*** refers to the absence of other causes or explanations.

• A ***temporal relationship*** must be determined. For example, the outcome must occur after the alleged cause.

• A ***biological gradient*** implies that higher or more frequent exposures increases the likelihood of the effect.

• ***Congruent data*** and epidemiologic relationships exist.

• Experiments to ***reproduce*** the effects also show a relationship.

• ***Analogous results*** help to reinforce possible causality. Sometimes this can be established by comparing similar exposures to similar effects.

While reviewing articles, common EBM terms are used. It is important to understand what each term means so that the information that is understood.

• ***Odds Ratio and Relative Risk (RR):*** A RR of 1.0 means that the exposure did not affect the outcome. An RR of 1.75 means that patients have a 75% increased risk of the outcome. An odds ratio is an estimate of relative risk when the RR cannot be calculated. Odd ratios are usually used in case-controlled studies.

• ***Clinical and statistical significance***: Statistical significance may not translate to clinical significance. In a way, it can be thought of as the difference between a disease-oriented outcome and a patient-oriented outcome. If a patient completes a questionnaire on depression and is one point away from a formal diagnosis of major depression, should the patient still be treated? In order for a study to show statistical significance, there must be enough patients in the study (referred to as the n). A study that enrolled 20 people is much less likely to show any statistical or clinical significance because the n is too small to represent the population at large.

• ***P value:*** A statistical measure, the P value helps to determine if a difference in an outcome between study groups happened by chance. A P of <.05 is considered valid.

• ***Confidence interval (CI):*** a statistical measure expressed as a range. If a study showed a 95% CI, it means that if the same study was repeated 100 times, the outcomes would still fall within the interval 95 times. A study that showed a diagnostic modality was 85% specific with a 95% CI of 80 – 90%, it means that if repeated 100 times, the specificity would fall between 80 – 90% 95 times. Narrow CIs are better.

• ***Intention-to-treat:*** An analysis of what happened to the study participants during the course of the study.

• ***Likelihood ratio (LR):*** A measure of the specificity or sensitivity of a test. An LR of 1.0 means that the probability of disease does not change. LRs should be high in order to rule in disease (generally considered >10), and LRs low (generally considered <0.1) to rule out disease.

• ***Number needed to treat (NNT):*** The number of patients who need to be treated to prevent one adverse outcome. Calculated with the ARR (1/ARR).

• ***Number needed to harm (NNH):*** The number of patients who need an intervention to prevent one adverse outcome.

• ***Absolute risk reduction (ARR):*** If the incidence of an adverse outcome in the control group is 20% and the incidence in the treatment group is 10%, then the ARR is 10% (20-10). Thus, the NNT would be 10 people (100% /ARR (100/10) in order to prevent one patient from experiencing an adverse outcome.

• ***Absolute risk increase (ARI):*** If the incidence of an adverse outcome is 2% in the treatment group, and the incidence of an adverse outcome is 1% in the control group, the NNH is 100 people (100%/(2% – 1%), and the ARI would be 1%.

• ***Predictive values,*** expressed as a percentage: A positive predictive value (PPV) is the percentage of people with a positive test who actually have a disease. Negative predictive value (NPV) is the percentage of people with a negative test who do not have a disease. Predictive values are reflections of how common or rare a disease presents in a population.

• ***Probability, Pre-test and Post-test:*** When a patient presents with a chief complaint, you are already working to develop a differential diagnosis list before you even begin the HPI. This is pre-test probability. After performing the history and physical examination, think about how likely a patient is to have a disease in your differential diagnoses. This is post-test probability. This can be a fluid process where differential diagnoses are up or down arrowed, depending on more information that is collected.

• ***Relative risk reduction (RRR):*** Expressed as a percentage of the difference between the control and treatment groups in outcomes. For example, if an adverse outcome occurs in 20% of the control group and 10% in the treatment group, there is a RRR of 50% ([20 − 10]/20)*100. If an adverse outcome occurred in 2% of the control group and 1% of the treatment group, there would still be a RRR of 50%, but would that difference be clinically significant? The ARR is more clinically significant because it subtracts the rates between the control group and the treatment group. Using the example above, in the first scenario, the ARR would be 10%, but in the second, it would only be 1%.

• ***Sensitivity:*** The ability of a test to correctly identify patients with a disease. Tests that are >95% sensitive mean that if the test is negative, you can safely rule out the presence of disease in that patient.

• ***Specificity:*** The ability of a test to correctly identify patients without a disease. Tests that are >95% specific mean that if the test is positive, you can safely rule in the presence of disease in that patient.

References:

1. OCEBM Levels of Evidence Working Group. The Oxford 2011 Levels of Evidence. Oxford Centre for Evidence-Based Medicine. http://www.cebm.net/index.aspx?o=5653

2. Hill AB. The environment and disease: association or causation? *Proc R Soc Med.* 1965;58(5):295-300.

3. EBM Glossary. American Family Physician. 2018. https://www.aafp.org/journals/afp/authors/ebm-toolkit/glossary.html

4. Sackett DL, Rosenberg WMC, Gray JAM, Haynes RB, Richardson WS. Evidence based medicine: what it is and what it isn't. *BMJ* 1996;312:71-2.

Identifying and Interpreting Data from Medical Informatics Sources and Identifying Appropriate Reference Sources

Medical information can come from various sources. **Primary sources** contain original research and are usually published in a scholarly, peer-reviewed journal. **Secondary sources** contain evaluations and reviews of primary research. Meta-analyses and systematic reviews are secondary sources. Review articles and review journals are also secondary sources. Most of the articles in the *Journal of the American Association of Physician Assistants* (JAAPA), for example, are secondary sources. Finally, **tertiary sources** combine primary and secondary sources into a reference format, such as a guidebook or encyclopedia.

Evaluating research findings by its quality of evidence is called grading. The gold standard for medicine is the GRADE system. GRADE stands for Grading of Recommendations Assessment, Development, and Evaluation. However, clinical practice guidelines utilize a different grading system. The United States Preventive Services Task Force (USPSTF) and the Agency for Healthcare Research and Quality (AHRQ) each use its own grading system. Below is a summary of the grading systems.

Grading of Recommendations Assessment, Development, and Evaluation (GRADE):

- **A:** The quality of evidence is **high**.
- **B:** The quality of evidence is **moderate**.
- **C:** The quality of evidence is **low**.
- **D:** The quality of evidence is **very low**.

Agency for Healthcare Research and Quality (AHRQ) practice guideline grading[1]:

- **A:** The research is good to support the recommendation.
- **B:** The research is fair to support the recommendation.
- **C:** The recommendation is based on clinical panel consensus and expert opinion.
- **X:** Evidence of harm exists for the intervention.

The United States Preventive Service Task Force (USPSTF) Guide to Clinical Preventive Services guideline grading[2]:

- **A:** There is high certainty that the benefit is strong, so offer the service.

- **B:** There is high certainty that the benefit is moderate to substantial, so offer the service.

- **C:** There is moderate certainty that there is a small benefit, and the evidence is insufficient to recommend offering or not offering the service.

- **D:** There is moderate to high certainty that there is no net benefit or there is harm, so do not offer the service.

- **I:** There is insufficient evidence to weight the benefits and harms, so if you offer the service, educate the patients about the conflict of evidence.

References:

1. The Agency for Healthcare Research and Quality. (2013). Grading the strength of a body of evidence when assessing healthcare interventions for the effective health care program of the Agency for Healthcare Research and Quality: An update. https://effectivehealthcare.ahrq.gov/topics/methods-guidance-grading-evidence/methods

2. United States Preventive Service Taskforce. Grade definitions. https://www.uspreventiveservicestaskforce.org/Page/Name/grade-definitions#grade-definitions-after-july-2012

POPULATION HEALTH, PUBLIC HEALTH[1,2,3]

Population health can be defined differently by various entities, and the definitions usually fit the specific population being treated. Population health seeks to improve health outcomes not just of the individual patient, but an entire population. Using data from health systems, both private and public, population health practitioners can identify and stratify patients within a population based upon specific risks. For example, one may examine a group of people with high risk diseases or conditions, people with rising risk, and people with low risk. The goal of population medicine is to: reduce the demand and need for health care resources through prevention strategies and patient education; reduce inappropriate use of resources; and increase the delivery of disease prevention and health promotion through quality improvement endeavors and collaborative relationships with public health and other community systems[4]. Population metrics also help to redefine guidelines. For example, research about the incidence and prevalence of cervical dysplasia in women under 21 years led to a new guideline that recommends against Pap testing in women under 21years.[5] In mid-2018, the American Cancer Society recommended that screening for colon cancer in average-risk patients begin at 45 instead of 50, a reflection of the increased rates of colon cancer in younger populations.[6]

Groups of people with high risk conditions tend to be high utilizers of medical services and usually experience worse health outcomes. People with rising risk may not have a high-risk condition, but through multi-disciplinary efforts may become low risk, thereby avoiding high utilization of health services and mitigating morbidity and mortality.

Multiple researchers have found that socioeconomic factors are the largest drivers of health and illness. Thus, population health considers the social determinants of health when analyzing data. PAs should also consider the type of environment in which patients live because those factors directly impact health outcomes.

Public health, on the other hand, seeks to protect and improve families and local and state communities through health promotion, screening, detection and treatment of infectious diseases, and injury prevention. However, population health is a discipline where public health, demography, and epidemiology merge with research on the social determinants of health to improved health outcomes. Prevention of illness and disease is central to public and population health.

The terms used to describe levels of prevention that you should know are:

• Primary prevention is an intervention that prevents the occurrence of an illness/disease. Classic examples of primary prevention are immunizations, tobacco cessation, and taking aspirin to help prevent preeclampsia.

> o *Changes in the social and physical environment where people live directly affect health outcomes. Primary preventive measures from a public health perspective also includes ensuring people live in asbestos-free and lead-free dwellings, have clean water to drink, and clean air to breathe.

• Secondary prevention is early detection of illness/disease through screening. Classic examples of secondary prevention are Pap testing and lipid monitoring.

> o *Public health clinics enable people to access immunizations and basic screening for disease.

• Tertiary prevention is an intervention that either delays or stops the progression of illness/disease. Classic examples of tertiary prevention include cardiac rehabilitation and screening for complications of disease.

> o *Public health workers can help to increase compliance with medications when patients are diagnosed with tuberculosis, for example, to decrease the risk of transmission to others and to help prevent drug resistance.

The AAFP developed a position paper on the importance of integrating public health concepts into patient care, and the IOM (now called the National Academy of Medicine) defined key competencies regarding training in population health science and public health. The IOM competencies are:

• *Population health:* knowledge of the fundamentals of population health, including a basic understanding of research; interdisciplinary skills that include the ability to lead and work with others; and knowledge exchange.

• *Public health:* knowledge of basic disaster preparedness; infection control measures/responses to outbreaks; occupational health issues for healthcare providers and non-healthcare workers; and travel health, population health, and epidemiology.

Do these competencies sound familiar? They should! These are all in the new 2019 NCCPA Professional Practice Blueprint.

Remember that one cannot separate an individual patient from the lived environment. A person's biology and psychology affect health outcomes, but so do other factors, such as the home, social network, work, indoor air, outside air, water, and even shifts in climate. Collectively called the social determinants of health, these are areas that directly and indirectly influence a person's health. Many federal agencies have begun to focus on the social determinants of health with evidence-based research that correlates these factors with morbidity and mortality rates, and ways to mitigate the effects. *Healthy People 2020* has focused on five areas of the social determinants of health:[7]

- Economic Stability: employment, food insecurity, housing instability, poverty

- Education: early childhood education and development, enrollment in higher education, high school graduation, language and literacy

- Social and Community Context: civic participation, discrimination, incarceration, social cohesion

- Health and Health Care: access to health care, access to primary care, health literacy

- Neighborhood and Built Environment: access to foods that support healthy eating patterns, crime and violence, environmental conditions, quality of housing

Healthy People 2020 supports initiatives that help to address the social determinants of health. For more information and resources, see: https://www.healthypeople.gov /2020/topics-objectives/topic/social-determinants-health/interventions-resources.

References:

1. What is public health? cdc.gov. http://www.cdcfoundation.org/content/what-public-health

2. Integration of Primary Care and Public Health (Position Paper). aafp.org. https://www.aafp.org/about/policies/all/integprimarycareandpublichealth.html

3. Training in Interdisciplinary Population Health Science: Current Successes and Future Needs. Bachrach C, et al. Executive Summary. http://www.healthandsocietyscholars.org/media/file/ExecSummTraining.pdf

4.   Horvath TV, Pomeranz H. Chapter 41: Population-based health. In Ballweg R, et al. *Physician Assistant: A Guide to Clinical Practice*. 5th ed. Philadelphia, PA: Elsevier; 2013.

5. Saslow D., et al. American Cancer Society, American Society for Colposcopy and Cervical Pathology, and American Society for Clinical Pathology screening guidelines for the prevention and early detection of cervical cancer. 2012. file:///C:/Users/elyse/Downloads/ASCCP%20Guidelines.pdf. Accessed on June 26, 2018.

6. American Cancer Society. Guideline for colorectal cancer screening for people at average risk. 2018. https://www.cancer.org/cancer/colon-rectal-cancer/detection-diagnosis-staging/acs-recommendations.html. Accessed on June 26, 2018.

7. Office of Disease Prevention and Health Promotion. *Healthy People 2020*: The social determinants of health. healthypeople.gov. https://www.healthypeople.gov/2020/topics-objectives/topic/social-determinants-of-health. Accessed on June 26, 2018.

BASIC PRINCIPLES OF EPIDEMIOLOGY[1,2]

Descriptive studies can be thought of as studies that determine person, place, and time of illness or disease. Are there certain occupations or people in a geographic region that seem to have the illness/disease? Does time of the year affect illness/disease? A descriptive study would not seek to test a hypothesis of etiology, for example, but it can provide important qualitative and quantitative data.

To discover the etiology of an illness/disease, an *analytic study* would provide the methodology to help with the discovery. For example, an analytic study might seek to find a common exposure among a population with the illness/disease. Unlike a descriptive study, an analytic study tests a hypothesis. An *experimental study* seeks to determine if an intervention mitigates or increases the risk of an illness/disease. In an experimental study, an intentional intervention occurs. In an *observational study*, researchers observe participants to determine if a variable affects an outcome without any intentional intervention. A *randomized controlled trial* is an example of an experimental study. Other types of analytic studies are *case-control and cohort*, but in these two study designs, the researcher does not intervene, thus, they are considered observational.

In every research study, one must consider the impact of potential *bias* on the study outcomes. Bias can be an error in the initial design of the study, the way in which the study was carried out, the way participants were selected, and the way in which data was analyzed. Bias can create an erroneous conclusion regarding risk of illness/disease, for example, if any systematic errors were made during the design, the execution, or the data analysis of the study. *Implicit bias* refers to unconscious negative attitudes about groups of people, often related to ethnicity/race, and can negatively affect research. Implicit bias can also negatively affect the way in which healthcare is delivered.[3]

Basic epidemiologic principles consider several metrics, such as *prevalence* and incidence. Prevalence is the number of cases of an illness/disease at a specified time divided by the population at risk. It is common to multiply this number by 100,000 to quantify a prevalence rate per 100,000 population. Incidence is the number of new cases of illness/disease that occurs over a specified period of time divided by the population at risk. This number is also multiplied by 100,000 to determine the incidence rate per 100,000 population.

The past several years has proven challenging to public health and disaster medicine as the U.S. and the world have dealt with Ebola virus, Zika virus, virulent influenza strains including Avian flu (H7N9) in China, Hepatitis A, E. coli, and even Plague in Madagascar. In the United States, there have been numerous food related outbreaks from Salmonella and E. coli in multiple food products, including lettuce, prepackaged cereals, and pre-cut fruit.4 There are several tools public health workers can use to estimate and predict the potential for an epidemic.[1] PAs also have a responsibility to report any unusual occurrence of a disease to the local health department.

The first step in predicting the potential for an epidemic is to define the *transmissibility* of the pathogen. An important measure of transmissibility is the (R0), or basic reproduction number. The (RO) is the number of secondary infections due to a single case. If the (R0>1), there is potential for an epidemic, but if the R0<1), there is no epidemic potential.

Another way public health workers and epidemiologists quantify a pathogen is through assessing its epidemic propensity by defining its *infectivity*, disease index, and virulence. The infectivity is the frequency of infection transmission between the susceptible person and the pathogen. The *disease index* is the number of people who develop disease divided by the total number of people infected. Virulence is the number of severe or fatal infections per total number of infections.

A pathogen should have a sufficient degree of infectivity to spread from person to person, sufficient virulence, and sufficient susceptibility of the host. Factors that can affect the host's susceptibility include age and immune status. Unfortunately, many infectious diseases that cause epidemics are associated with malnutrition, poverty, and war. Other conditions that can predispose to epidemics are overcrowding, contaminated water, and chronic stress among populations.

Recognizing an epidemic and the causative pathogen is the first step towards controlling it. Once the pathogen has been determined, the *route of transmission* needs to be determined. Control of the spread of the illness/disease must occur through various methodologies including isolating carriers, immunizing populations at risk, using chemoprophylaxis when appropriate, blocking transmission, and rectifying contaminated areas.

An *emerging infectious disease* is defined as an illness/disease that is reappearing and increasing in incidence or is expected to increase in the near future. Often, these pathogens have been around for many years, but due to mutations or resistance patterns, they have different characteristics that may be difficult to treat. Sometimes an emerging infectious disease is a newly identified pathogen, and sometimes it is an old pathogen with a new geographic distribution or mutation.

There are various factors that are associated with the emergence or reemergence of infectious diseases. These include changing demographics, particularly human movement into habitats that have previously been occupied by animals; irrigation systems that fail to address pathogen colonization; ease of international travel; fractures in public health systems that lead to disruptions in sanitation; ecologic changes; and antibiotic drug resistance. It is important to remember that all of these issues occur on a global scale.

Antimicrobial resistance is widely acknowledged as a public health threat. Currently, resistance to multiple drugs are seen with Clostridium difficile, carbapenem-resistant Enterobacteriaceae, methicillin resistant Staphylococcus aureus, and Neisseria gonorrhoeae2. Extremely drug-resistant pathogens are also of significant concern. Extremely drug-resistant tuberculosis occurs in almost all parts of the world, including the U.S.

Reemerging pathogens include Measles, Lyme disease, Listeriosis, drug-resistant Malaria, Dengue, Yellow fever, Zika virus, Adenovirus 14, Plague, Diphtheria, Ebola virus, West Nile virus, Typhoid fever, Chikungunya, and Cholera.

Newly emerging pathogens include Hantavirus pulmonary syndrome, E. coli O157:H7 and O104:H4, Enterovirus D68, Cryptosporidiosis, Severe acute respiratory

All PAs should apprise themselves of new information regarding epidemics, pandemics, reemerging, and newly emerging infectious diseases. When your local health department sends notices, it is wise to pay attention to what is happening locally. However, pay attention to what is happening globally as well.

References:

1. Chapter 5: Emerging and Reemerging Infectious Diseases: Emergence and Global Spread of Infection. In Ryan KJ, ed. Sherris Medical Microbiology, 7e. New York: McGraw-Hill. http://accessmedicine.mhmedical.com/content.aspx?bookid=2268&sectionid=176081144. Accessed on May 16, 2018.

2. Paules CI, Eisinger RW, Marston HD, Fauci AS. What recent history has taught us about responding to emerging infectious disease threats. Ann Intern Med. 2017;167:805-811.

3. FitzGerald C, Hurst S. Implicit bias in healthcare professionals: A review. *BMC Med Ethics*. 2017; 18: 19. Published online 2017 Mar 1. doi: 10.1186/s12910-017-0179-8.

4. Centers for Disease Control and Prevention. List of selected multistate foodborne outbreak investigations. cdc.gov. https://www.cdc.gov/foodsafety/outbreaks/multistate-outbreaks/outbreaks-list.html. Accessed on June 26, 2018.

TRAVEL HEALTH[1]

Patients will often seek advice from their PAs regarding immunizations and medications needed or suggested prior to international travel. Local public health departments will often be the suppliers of immunizations that are required for international travel, such as Yellow Fever vaccination. The CDC posts notices regarding travel to international countries using a 3-level warning system.

- Warning Level 3: AVOID nonessential travel

- Alert Level 2: Use enhanced precautions

- Watch Level 1: Use the usual precautions

For up-to-date country-specific information about safety and security, see the U.S. Department of State Travel Advisories page: https://travel.state.gov/content/travel/en/traveladvisories/traveladvisories.html

The CDC offers a guidebook on international travel. Referred to as the Yellow Book, it is updated and published every two years with update about emerging and reemerging infectious diseases, new vaccination recommendations, and guidance regarding the use of antimicrobials. You can purchase the book at: https://wwwnc.cdc.gov/travel/page/yellowbook-home.

Malaria[1]

Malaria is perhaps one of the most commonly encountered diseases when traveling overseas to endemic areas. While there are medications to help prevent infection, the CDC recommends all travels still use mosquito avoidance measures, such as Environmental Protection Agency (EPA)-approved insect repellent, long pants and long sleeves, and with an insecticide-treated bednet.

The CDC suggests asking the following questions when determining risk of malaria transmission:

1. To where is the patient going?

a. If an area has sporadic malaria cases and the risk of infection to people is considered very low, patients should use mosquito avoidance measures but no medication prophylaxis.

b. If an area has a high risk of infection to people, medication prophylaxis plus mosquito avoidance measures should be used.

c. Always consult the CDC's website on malaria transmission by country at: https://wwwnc.cdc.gov/travel/yellowbook/2018/infectious-diseases-related-to-travel/malaria#5217

2. When is the patient traveling?

a. Malaria transmission can vary by season. Again, consult the CDC website above.

3. For what purpose is the patient traveling?

a. Ask about the type of accommodations and if the patient is going to spend time outdoors, particularly at night as mosquitos are more active at night. A patient who is spending a short time in an air-conditioned hotel will probably have a lower chance of malaria transmission than if camping or staying in primitive housing.

4. How long will the patient be in the country?

a. Longer stays mean a higher likelihood of exposure.

5. Who is traveling?

a. Some people are known to have a greater likelihood of malaria transmission, such as pregnant women. Infection with malaria during pregnancy can result in significant risks to the fetus and mother, including abortion, fetal death, and prematurity.

b. The highest risk is actually 1st and 2nd generation US immigrants who are traveling back to their native malaria-endemic countries. These patients should receive medication prophylaxis and practice mosquito avoidance measures.

The CDC also recommends use of the following the Environmental Protection Agency's registered mosquito repellants while traveling to endemic Malaria (and Zika virus) countries that are safe even in pregnancy and lactation:

• N, N-Diethyl-meta-toluamide (DEET)

• Picaridin (known as KBR 3023 and icaridin outside the US)

• IR3535

• Oil of lemon eucalyptus (OLE) or para-menthane-diol (PMD)

• 2-undecanone

For all antimalarials, it is best to contact the CDC's website to verify resistance patterns in the area your patient is traveling. Common drugs used in malaria prophylaxis include:

• Atovaquone/Proguanil (Malarone): start 1-2 days before travel, take daily and continue for 7 days upon return. Not for use in pregnancy or breastfeeding infants or in severe renal impairment.

• Chloroquine: Taken weekly and started 1 – 2 weeks before travel, continue for four weeks upon return. Safe in pregnancy. Not for use in areas with chloroquine or mefloquine resistance.

• Doxycycline: start 1 – 2 days before travel, take daily and continue for 4 weeks upon return. Not for use in pregnancy.

• Mefloquine (Lariam): Taken weekly and started 1 – 2 weeks before travel, continue for 4 weeks upon return. Safe for use in pregnancy. Not for use if mefloquine resistance is present, in patients with psychiatric diseases, seizure disorders, and cardiac conduction abnormalities. Can cause nightmares.

• Primaquine: best choice for preventing P. vivax. Taken daily, start 1 – 2 days before travel, and continue for 7 days upon return. Not for use in patients with G6PD deficiency, pregnant, or breastfeeding women.

Reference:

1. Centers for Disease Control and Prevention. Chapter 3: Infectious Diseases Related to Travel. 2018. cdc.gov. https://wwwnc.cdc.gov/travel/yellowbook /2018/infectious-diseases-related-to-travel/malaria#5217

Zika virus[1]

Zika virus can cause significant birth defects in infected pregnant women. The CDC advises that pregnant women, women who are trying to conceive, and the partners of women trying to conceive do not travel to Zika-endemic areas.

Travelers to Zika-endemic areas should avoid mosquito bites for three weeks after return to the U.S. so that if a mosquito bites the traveler, the mosquito will not transmit the virus to others.

For information on Zika, visit https://wwwnc.cdc.gov/travel/page/zika-information

Reference:

1. Centers for Disease Control and Prevention. Zika virus. 2018. cdc.org. https://www.cdc.gov/zika/index.html

Cholera[1]

The Advisory Committee on Immunization Practices recommends that people age 18 – 64 years traveling to Vibrio cholerae endemic areas receive an oral, single-dose cholera vaccine (CVD 103-HgR, Vaxchora [PaxVax Corporation, Redwood City, CA]). The CDC recommends that while cholera in travelers is quite rare, PAs and other emergency responders who travel to areas with active cholera for humanitarian relief, and others who plan on prolonged visits, receive the vaccine. However, water and food precautions and hand hygiene are perhaps the most important prevention.

The CDC regularly updates their websites regarding travel to foreign countries. Fifteen countries in Africa are on the list; in Asia, Bangladesh, India, and Yemen; and Haiti in the Americas.

Reference:

1. Clinical update: Cholera vaccine for travelers. cdc.gov. https://wwwnc.cdc.gov/travel/news-announcements/cholera-vaccine-for-travelers

Polio[1]

Wild poliovirus emerged as a public health emergency in 2014, so the World Health Organization updated polio vaccination recommendations. If patients plan on staying more than four weeks in Nigeria, Pakistan, or Afghanistan, they must be prepared to show proof of polio vaccination when they leave the respective countries. As such, people who plan on staying for more than four weeks in one of these countries must plan on being vaccinated with a dose of inactivated polio vaccine (IPV) or bivalent oral polio vaccine (bOPV) between four weeks and twelve months BEFORE their departure from these countries.

It is also recommended that documentation of polio vaccination on the International Certificate of Vaccination or Prophylaxis (found here: https://bookstore.gpo.gov/products/international-certificate-vaccination-or-prophylaxis-approved-world-health-organization-0).

If a patient requires urgent travel and has not had a dose of IPV within the previous four weeks to 12 months, the patient should receive a dose of polio vaccine. Adults should receive a polio vaccine booster if they have already completed the polio vaccination series. If their polio status is unknown or incomplete, they should receive two doses with 1 – 2 months between doses, and a third dose 6 – 12 months after the second dose.

Infants and children who have completed their polio vaccination series, but received the last dose more than 12 months prior should have another dose of IPV.

Reference:

1. Clinical Update: Interim CDC Guidance for Travel to and from Countries Affected by the New Polio Vaccine Requirements. cdc.gov. https://wwwnc.cdc.gov/travel/news-announcements/polio-guidance-new-requirements

Yellow fever

Yellow fever is endemic in tropical South American (particularly Brazil) and sub-Saharan Africa. The illness occurs through the bite of mosquito infected with the virus. However, humans who are infected with the virus can transmit the virus to a mosquito who then can transmit it to another human. Perinatal transmission has also been documented.

Symptoms of Yellow fever mimic influenza, with fever, chills, myalgias, back pain, and headaches. A subset of infected patients can develop severe disease that can be fatal. The CDC recommends travelers to endemic areas be vaccinated with Yellow fever vaccine at least 10 days prior to travel, but should also practice mosquito avoidance.

Reference:

1. Yellow Fever. cdc.gov. 2018. https://wwwnc.cdc.gov/travel/yellowbook/2018/infectious-diseases-related-to-travel/yellow-fever

Traveler's diarrhea[1]

The most common cause of traveler's diarrhea is bacteria, including *enterotoxigenic Escherichia coli*, *Campylobacter jejuni*, and *Salmonella* and *Shigella* species. Viral etiologies include rotavirus, norovirus, and astovirus. The most common protozoal etiology is *Giardia lamblia*. The areas associated with the highest risk of traveler's diarrhea include Mexico, Central America, South American, parts of Asia, the Middle East, and Africa.

Traveler's diarrhea due to bacteria usually develops within a few hours, and protozoal infections can sometimes take up to two weeks to become symptomatic. Mild to moderate traveler's diarrhea due to bacterial etiologies tend to resolve on their own within one week, while viral etiologies resolve within 2 -3 days. Protozoal etiologies can have an incubation period up to two weeks and can persist for months if untreated.

Treatment of mild traveler's diarrhea on patients > 6 years using an antimotility medication and no antibiotic may be appropriate, but oral rehydration is always first-line. Bismuth subsalicylate is recommended for traveler's diarrhea unless the patient is < 3 years old; pregnant; has an allergy to aspirin; has renal insufficiency and/or gout; and/or taking methotrexate, probenecid, or anticoagulants.

Remember that anti-motility medications should be avoided if the patient has bloody diarrhea and/or fever. In patients with moderate to severe traveler's diarrhea, a fluoroquinolone or azithromycin can be used, but fluoroquinolone resistance is increasing. Infection with Giardia can be treated with metronidazole or tinidazole.

Reference:

1. Connor BA. Chapter 2. The Pretravel Consultation: Traveler's diarrhea. cdc.gov. 2018. https://wwwnc.cdc.gov/travel/yellowbook/2018/the-pre-travel-consultation/travelers-diarrhea

OCCUPATIONAL HEALTH

PAs can be primarily employed in occupational health clinics but may also see occupational health patients in urgent care centers and emergency departments. Some PAs work specifically for an employer and thus must disclose this to the patient. PAs can provide medical screenings for the Department of Transportation through the Federal Motor Carrier Safety Administration (FMCSA) by completing required training, registering to be a licensed medical examiner through the FMCSA, and passing a national exam, called the National Registry Medical Examiner certification test.

Issues related to occupational health and illness can arise in almost all healthcare settings and are not limited to healthcare workers. For example, it is estimated that there are over three million migrant farmworkers in the U.S. at any given time.[1] Migrant farmworkers are at substantial risk of occupational illnesses, injuries, and other diseases. Common illnesses include respiratory and skin exposure illness due to pesticide and other chemical exposures; traumatic injuries; infectious diseases; and musculoskeletal injuries.[2] According to the EPA there are 20,000 medical provider diagnosed pesticide poisonings each year among farmworkers in the U.S. It is recommended that agricultural and migrant farmworkers are asked the following questions to ascertain risk:

- Do you know of any pesticides that are being used at work and/or at home?

- When picking fruits/vegetables, are the fields wet or dry?

- Are you aware of any spraying while you were working?

- Do you receive notification of when spraying will occur?

- Have you had any safety training?

- How do you feel during and after work?

- Do you experience eye problems or skin problems during or after work?

- Can you shower or bathe and change into clean clothes after work?

Other populations are at risk for developing asthma and other respiratory diseases due to occupational exposure. Some of these populations include anyone working with animals; hair stylists and nail salon workers; and painters, particularly if using spray paint. In addition, workers from minority groups and lower socioeconomic status are at greater risk of experiencing work injuries.

While performing a social history, ask about a patient's occupation and follow up with questions about occupational risk. It is helpful to try and asses overall risk by asking the following questions:[2]

• Do you think your symptoms/illness/disease are related to work?

• Do your symptoms improve when you are not at work?

• Do you know if you have ever been exposed to any chemicals at work, including dust, chemicals, radiation, and even persistent loud noise?

• Do you use personal protective equipment and have you been trained on safety?

If a patient is identified as having experienced an occupational exposure to a hazardous material, documentation and prompt consultation are imperative. If unaware of the harm potential, call the local poison-control center. Most health systems will have a separate electronic health system or paperwork for work-related injuries. A worker who is injured or becomes ill due to a work-related issue may be eligible for worker's compensation.

Many PAs specialize in occupational medicine and can become members of The American Academy of Physician Assistants in Occupational Medicine (AAPA-OM). The AAPA, the American College of Occupational and Environmental Medicine, and the National Institute for Occupational Safety and Health offer specific CME in occupational medicine and even provide avenues for certification in providing Department of Transportation physical examinations through the FMCSA.

References:

1. Demographics. National Center for Farmworker Health, Inc. http://www.ncfh.org/uploads/3/8/6/8/38685499/fs-migrant_demographics.pdf. Accessed on 5/17/2018.

2. Guarnieri M, Diaz JV, Balmes JR. Chapter 25: Work, living environment, and health. In Medical Management of Vulnerable and Underserved Patients: Principles, Practice, and Populations, 2e. McGraw-Hill Lange; 2016.

Resources:

American Academy of PAs in Occupational Medicine:
http://www.aapaoccmed.org/

Federal Motor Carrier Safety Administration:
https://www.fmcsa.dot.gov/regulations/medical/national-registry-certified-medical-examiners-become-certified-medical-examiner

The National Institute for Occupational Safety and Health:
http://www.cdc.gov/niosh/topics/

The World Health Organization: http://www.euro.who.int/en/health-topics/environment-and-health

The U.S. Environmental Protection Agency's National Strategies for Health Care Providers: Pesticide Initiative.
http://www.epa.gov/oppfead1/safety/healthcare/handbook/handbook.pdf;
http://www.epa.gov/pesticides/safety/healthcare/healthcare.htm.

NEEDLESTICK INJURIES IN HEALTHCARE WORKERS[1]

Approximately 800,000 needlestick injuries occur in the US annually[1]. Safer devices have been developed to help decrease the risk of a needlestick injury but it is still important to become familiar with the devices and always be vigilant about handling any sharp instrument.

If a needlestick or sharp injury occurs and there is a possibility of blood or body fluid exposure, one must:

• Use soap and water to wash the injury.

• Copiously flush and irrigate the skin, nose, mouth, and eyes if blood or body fluids are splashed.

• Report the injury to the immediate supervisor and any other required personnel.

• Seek medical treatment.

Postexposure prophylaxis (PEP) aims to treat possible exposure to HIV with antiretroviral therapy.

• If there is any suspicion about possible HIV exposure, PEP is recommended. The HIV status of the patient, while helpful, is not necessary to begin PEP.

• PEP should begin as soon as possible with three or more antiretroviral medications.

• The preferred medications are tenofovir (tenofovir DF or TDF) with emtricitabine plus raltegravir.

• The first follow-up exam should occur within 72 hours of the injury/exposure.

• Follow-up includes testing for HIV and drug toxicity should occur at baseline, at six weeks, 12 weeks, and six months.

• If a combination of HIV p24 antigen-HIV antibody test is used, testing can conclude four months after the initial exposure; otherwise, testing should conclude after six months.

Nonoccupational postexposure prophylaxis (nPEP) for HIV[2]

When patients present ≤ 72 hours after a possible HIV exposure, PAs should evaluate the patient for nPEP candidacy. Patients should have a rapid HIV serology test, but if a rapid test is unavailable and the patient is considered a candidate for nPEP, antiviral therapy should be initiated. The preferred regimen is triple-therapy for 28 days. The preferred medications are tenofovir (tenofovir DF or TDF) with emtricitabine plus raltegravir or dolutegravir. If the patient presents >72 hours after exposure, nPEP is not recommended. In patients with risk factors for HIV, such as intravenous drug use and sex work, appropriate counseling should occur with consideration for preexposure prophylaxis.

If patients present >72 hours after exposure; are pregnant or breastfeeding; had contact with someone known to be antiretroviral-resistant; and/or have serious co-morbidities, infectious disease consultation is recommended.

Hepatitis C[3]

If healthcare workers present with a needlestick or body fluid exposure and Hepatitis C is suspected, the healthcare worker should be tested for anti-HCV within 48 hours of the exposure.

If the patient tests positive, order a reflex HCV RNA test. If the reflex HCV RNA test is positive, the patient is considered to have preexisting Hepatitis C and should be referred appropriately.

If the patient tests negative for anti-HCV, repeat testing at least three weeks after the exposure is recommended. If repeat testing is negative, no further testing is required. If the patient tests positive, refer as appropriate.

Hepatitis B[4]

Healthcare workers who experience a potential exposure to Hepatitis B should have their immune status verified. If the healthcare worker is immune, no further testing or vaccination is required. If the healthcare worker is a non-responder (defined as having anti-HBs <10mIU/mL after at least six doses of Hepatitis B vaccine) and the status of the source is positive or unknown, administer Hepatitis B immune globulin (HBIG) as soon as possible and again in one month. If the healthcare worker's response to vaccination is <10mIU/mL and the status of the source is positive or unknown, HBIG is administered for one dose only and restart the Hepatitis B vaccination series. If the status of the source is negative, there is no recommendation to administer HBIG, but restarting the Hepatitis B vaccination series is recommended. If the healthcare worker is unvaccinated, incompletely vaccinated, or refuses vaccination and the source is positive or unknown, HBIG is recommended as soon as possible.

References:

1. How to prevent needlestick injuries. osha.gov. https://www.osha.gov/Publications/osha3161.pdf. Accessed on 5/17/208.

2. Updated guidelines for antiretroviral postexposure prophylaxis after sexual, injection drug use, or other nonoccupational exposure to HIV—United States, 2016 April 18, 2016 https://stacks.cdc.gov/view/cdc/38856

3. Kuhar DT, et al. Updated US Public Health Service Guidelines for the Management of Occupational Exposures to Human Immunodeficiency Virus and Recommendations for Postexposure Prophylaxis. Infect Control Hosp *Epidemiol*. 2013 Sep;34(9):875-92. doi: 10.1086/672271. http://www.jstor.org/stable/pdf/10.1086/672271.pdf?refreqid=excelsior%3A8d3981ecd2a584270e9516dddbdb70cf

4. Information for Healthcare Personnel Potentially Exposed to Hepatitis C Virus (HCV). cdc.gov. https://www.cdc.gov/hepatitis/pdfs/Testing-Followup-Exposed-HC-Personnel.pdf. Accessed on 5/18/2018.

5. CDC Guidance for Evaluating Health-Care Personnel for Hepatitis B Virus Protection and for Administering Postexposure Management. *Recommendations and Reports* December 20, 2013 / 62(RR10);1-19. https://www.cdc.gov/mmwr/preview/mmwrhtml/rr6210a1.htm. Accessed on 5/18/2018.

Resources:

Clinician's Postexposure Prophylaxis (PEP) hotline: 888-448-4911 or http://www.nccc.ucsf.edu/

BASIC DISASTER PREPAREDNESS

Medical disaster response in the U.S, has closely followed models from the military where much information has been gained regarding how to manage mass casualty scenarios, particularly in high-stress environments where supplies may be lacking. It has been argued that while this type of model works well in battle settings, it does not always work well when a natural disaster or man-made disaster occurs on domestic soil. As such, disaster medicine has become a medical specialty wherein PAs can gain formal training in disaster preparedness, policy, and response. Many PAs volunteer or work on disaster medical assistance teams and respond to federal and international disasters.

The Joint Commission requires hospitals to hold two disaster drills annually[1]. These drills help to keep healthcare providers and staff familiar with procedures, roles, and responsibilities if a disaster occurred. The extent of the drill is up to the facility and can range from computer-based scenarios, mini-drills, and large-scale simulations.

When disasters strike, the PA and all other responders must be adaptive to the new challenges that will occur. Disaster medicine requires integrated processes where medical responders rely on other specialists to carry out an efficient response. Hendrickson and Horowitz[1] outlined a plan for responding to a disaster. Following these steps can assist disaster preparedness groups in planning for and responding to a disaster.

- Activate the emergency operations plan.

- Establish an emergency operations center (also called an Incident Command Post).

- Quickly assess hospital/facility capacity.

    o Hospitals should know how many casualties can be managed at each location

- Create surge capacity (increasing capacity over normal numbers).

    o Can include placing multiple patients in a room, converting non-patient rooms to areas where care can be provided, and utilizing nonemergency spaces for acute patient care.

- Establish communications with all stakeholders.

- Inventory supplies.

- o The CDC can restock certain supplies during a disaster within 12 hours. http://www.bt.cdc.gov/stockpile/index.asp

- Establish and maintain support areas.

- Designate areas of the facility for triage, treatment, and decontamination.

   - o Triage requires the rapid assessment of patients with dispersal to the appropriate treatment areas

   - o Treatment should be divided into different areas based upon the severity of the patient.

      - Seriously ill and injured patients are sent to the resuscitation area and surgical candidates are sent to a presurgical holding area or surgical triage

      - The number of operating rooms is the limiting factor in caring for trauma victims in massive disasters

      - Minor illnesses and injuries are sent to a low acuity area

- Designate an area for mental health assessment and treatment.

- Designate an area as a morgue.

During the acute phase, or the first 24 hours, it is important to make sure roles are defined and communication is open. An integrated response with emergency medical services, behavioral medicine providers, fire and law enforcement, public health agencies, volunteer organizations, local businesses, and academic institutions can yield better outcomes that siloed or fragmented responses.

During the immediate response time, or the first two hours, find out if an Incident Command Post (ICP) has been set up. If so, who is the Incident Commander (IC)and how do you communicate with him or her? Find out if infrastructure has been affected, such as electrical, water, and sanitation. The intermediate response time is between six and 12 hours after the disaster. The CDC recommends that as communication with the public during this time is critical, it is prudent to prepare messaging that uses the STARCC Principle as developed by Reynolds in 2004[2].

S: Simple. People who are scared need basic information in a way they can understand it.

T: Timely. People want the information right away.

A: Accurate. Provide information that is truthful.

R: Relevant. Answer any questions and provide information that is appropriate to the circumstance.

C: Credible. Convey empathy and openness while maintaining professionalism and credibility.

C: Consistent. Any change in messaging from one press conference, statement, or directive can cause confusion and chaos.

The extended response occurs between 12 – 24 hours. This may be the time when members of the public health team start collecting and analyzing data. Be aware of responder fatigue and address any concerns with the team leader or Incident Commander. This is also a good time to take inventory of supplies to make sure care can continue to be provided.

While every PA, despite area of practice, can be trained in disaster medicine preparedness, emergency medicine PAs must have knowledge of the processes and basic principles of disaster medicine. Training for PAs can be accomplished through several organizations. The Department of Health and Human Services' National Disaster Medical System offers membership, training, volunteer opportunities, and paid positions in their organization. More information can be found here: https://www.phe.gov/Preparedness/responders/ndms/Pages/default.aspx.

The CDC recommends that medical responders have, at minimum, updated tetanus and Hepatitis B immunization for domestic responses. Other immunizations may be appropriate depending upon the situation and location of response.

Basic infection control measures aim to prevent water-borne illnesses and respiratory diseases. Hand washing is still perhaps the most important intervention during a disaster or outbreak, and personal protective equipment, including masks and gloves, should be used judiciously. The CDC has guidelines regarding the identification of treatment of certain respiratory and diarrheal illnesses common during disasters and outbreaks and can be found here: https://www.cdc.gov/disasters/infectioncontrol.html. Comprehensive information on infection control and health and safety during and after natural disasters can be found here: https://www.cdc.gov/disasters/alldisasters.html.

The CDC also offers continuing medical education, training, newsletters, conference calls, and webinars for healthcare providers who are involved in, or wish to become involved in disaster medicine and preparedness. The Clinician Outreach and Communication Activity (COCA) is the arm of the CDC tasked to prepare healthcare providers to respond appropriately to mass emergencies, public health threats, disease outbreaks, terrorism, and natural disasters. For more information, visit: https://emergency.cdc.gov/coca/about.asp.

Preparing your patients for potential disasters is encouraged, particularly if you practice in a location known to experience natural disasters, such as tornadoes, hurricanes, and floods. The CDC recommends that at a minimum, the following items should be included in an easily accessible kit[3].

- Clean water. One gallon per person per day for at least three days.

- Canned foods or nonperishable foods.

- Bedding items, including blankets and pillows.

- Battery operated radio (or solar or hand-crank)

- Extra batteries of various sizes

- Flashlights

- A first aid kit

- Essential medications

- At least one multipurpose device to use a tool

- Hygiene and sanitation products

- Extra clothing appropriate for different temperatures

- Bleach

- Duct tape

- Plastic tarps

- Matches

Ask patients if they have developed an emergency plan for their families. All emergency numbers should be either posted somewhere obvious or readily available. Identify two meeting places, one close to home and one further away in case access to the home is limited. Have an escape route planned for each member of the family.

References:

1. Chapter 5: Disaster Preparedness. Hendrickson RG, Horowitz, BZ. In: Tintinalli JE, Stapczynski J, Ma O, Yeagly DM, Meckler GD, Cline DM. eds. Tintitalli's Emergency Medicine: A Comprehensive Study Guide, 8e. New York: McGray-Hill; 2016.http://accessmedicine.mhmedical.com/content.aspx?bookid=1658 &sectionid=109381281. Accessed 5/16/2018.

2. Reynolds, B., Crisis and Emergency Risk Communication by Leaders for Leaders. Atlanta, GA: Centers for Disease Control and Prevention, 2004

3. Petersen M, Allison LG. Chapter 52: Mass casualty and disaster management. In Ballweg R, et al. Physician Assistant: A Guide to Clinical Practice. 5th ed. Philadelphia, PA: Elsevier; 2013.

Bibliography:

About COCA. cdc.org. https://emergency.cdc.gov/coca/about.asp

Ciottone GR, et al. Introduction to disaster medicine. In Ciottone's Disaster Medicine (2nd Ed);2016. Philadelphia, PA: Elsevier

Emergency planners and responders. Cdc.gov. https://emergency.cdc.gov/planners-responders.asp. Accessed 5/18/2018

Guidelines for the Management of Acute Diarrhea After a Disaster. cdc.gov.https://www.cdc.gov/disasters/infectioncontrol.html

Public Health Emergency Response Guide for State, Local, and Tribal Public Health Directors Version 2.0. April 2011. cdc.gov. https://emergency.cdc.gov/planning/pdf/cdcresponseguide.pdf. Accessed 5/13/2018.

OTHER RESOURCES THAT MAY BE OF INTEREST AND VALUE TO THE PA

Emergency Responder Health Monitoring and Surveillance (ERHMS) Course

The National Disaster Life Support Foundation (www.ndls.net)

Strategic National Stockpile Training and Exercises

Environmental Health Training in Emergency Response

Reproductive Health in Emergency Preparedness and Response

https://emergency.cdc.gov/planning/medcon/index.asp

https://emergency.cdc.gov/epix/index.asp

https://www.cdc.gov/phpr/readiness/mcm.html

ABOUT THE AUTHOR

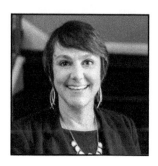

Elyse Watkins, DHSc, PA-C, DFAAPA earned her Doctor of Health Science in December 2016 with a focus on global health from Nova Southeastern University. She is a graduate of The George Washington University's PA program in 1993 and has been a practicing PA since then.

The majority of Dr. Watkins clinical work has been in ob/gyn and primary care. She has spent the past six years in PA education teaching across the curriculum, including courses in evidence based medicine and health care policy and ethics. She has spoken at multiple state PA conferences and at AAPA, has had numerous articles published in JAAPA, and has been an invited author for several books.

CPSIA information can be obtained
at www.ICGtesting.com
Printed in the USA
BVHW090729140519
548198BV00003B/6/P